SUBSTITUTE
Yourself
Skinny

Chef SUSAN IRBY
the Bikini Chef

adamsmedia
Avon, Massachusetts

Published by
Adams Media, a division of F+W Media, Inc.
57 Littlefield Street, Avon, MA 02322. U.S.A.
www.adamsmedia.com

ISBN 10: 1-4405-0397-4
ISBN 13: 978-1-4405-0397-9

Printed in China

10   9   8   7   6   5   4   3   2   1

Library of Congress Cataloging-in-Publication Data
is available from the publisher.

This publication is designed to provide accurate and authoritative information with regard to the subject matter covered. It is sold with the understanding that the publisher is not engaged in rendering legal, accounting, or other professional advice. If legal advice or other expert assistance is required, the services of a competent professional person should be sought.
—From a *Declaration of Principles* jointly adopted by a Committee of the American Bar Association and a Committee of Publishers and Associations

Many of the designations used by manufacturers and sellers to distinguish their product are claimed as trademarks. Where those designations appear in this book and Adams Media was aware of a trademark claim, the designations have been printed with initial capital letters.

Calorieking.com was used to calculate the nutritional values for these recipes.

All interior photos by Albert Evangelista, except as noted:
Page 10 © istockphoto / robynmac
Page 47 © istockphoto / wsmahar
Page 79 © istockphoto / tovfla
Page 109 © istockphoto / toulouse_lulu
Page 178 © StockFood / Shaffer-Smith
Page 226 © StockFood / Milne

This book is available at quantity discounts for bulk purchases.
For information, please call 1-800-289-0963.

acknowledgments

Thank you to the talented, patient, supportive professionals at Adams Media: Chelsea, Laura, the Adams production team . . . without you this book would not have been possible. To my remarkable agent, Uwe Stender, who believed in The Bikini Chef. Thank you to my friend, Denice Fladeboe, and Fladeboe Automotive Group of Irvine for your constant support. To my husband, Christopher Moore, for putting up with our home becoming a photography studio and for calming my nerves when I thought I would go crazy.

Thanks to Sue Recker, Lauren Moore, and my daughter-by-marriage, Rachel. And finally, to my mother, Melba, who turned her Alabama home into a cookbook-writing workshop and spent endless hours helping me with this book and testing recipes, and to my longtime friend, Celeste, who joined us.

contents

thinner dinners
73

deliciously skinny desserts
187

index
228

introduction

Eating healthy meals can feel like a constant battle. My whole life I have strived to find a balance between staying slim and trim and enjoying the fattening foods I love. We all have our high-calorie favorites, our "comfort" foods—lasagna, tacos, fettuccini Alfredo—and then the desserts . . . cheesecake, triple chocolate cake, or "pack-on-the-pounds" pound cake. They taste so good, you just have to *have* them. You don't want to feel left out when everyone else is enjoying lasagna and you're eating humdrum cottage cheese and tomatoes!

For all the satisfaction you may get out of eating high-calorie foods, what is not satisfying is how overly full and heavy you often feel afterward. How often do you see the leftover (full of sugar) strawberry pie from your dinner out or chocolate brownies you made for a party and think, "Oh, I'll just eat one bite?" You stand over the sink and eat one bite, then two bites, then another bite, and before you know it, you've eaten the whole dessert! We've all been there. After that, if you are like me, you end up feeling fat, depressed, and your energy is zapped. Those are not fun feelings to have and that's no way to spend your life . . . spinning your wheels worrying about what you eat or don't eat. It doesn't have to be this way!

If you can relate to these feelings, then *Substitute Yourself Skinny* can help you. The simple truth is that the only way to break the negative/unhealthy/overindulging/fattening food cycle is to replace overly fattening foods with less-fattening foods that taste as good or better than the overly fattening foods! This book is all about substitutions that still taste good, and even taste better!

As a "foodie" who likes to look good too, I have put together 175 recipes and "Skinny Secret" tricks to help you eat more sensibly while still enjoying the foods you love. And, these recipes are not bland, "diet" foods—they are your favorite, fattening foods made lighter, fresher, healthier, and flavorful.

And, to be as helpful as possible, I have included calorie counts for the original high-calorie recipe, the lower-calorie *Substitute Yourself Skinny* recipe, and calculated your calorie savings per serving! Right away, you will be able to see the calories you saved per serving by cooking up the lower-calorie, high-flavor version of the recipes you love. This allows you to track daily how many calories you have saved, which add up to losing those unwanted pounds! In addition, you'll find the recipe's fat, carbohydrates, protein, and sodium counts. These numbers will help you maintain a healthy overall diet packed with nutrients.

Let's get started!

the skinny on substitutions

Mention the word "substitution" in relation to a recipe and people get a little nervous—afraid their food is going to taste funny and have an odd texture if they nix their favorite, traditional high-fat ingredients for a lower-calorie counterpart. Substituting healthier, lower-calorie foods just doesn't always sound so appealing. But that's where *Substitute Yourself Skinny* comes in! This book will help you turn your favorite high-calorie foods into lower-calorie favorites you can enjoy every day, guilt-free!

Let's face it: Our culinary world has changed from when our parents and grandparents began cooking. Reduced-fat and nonfat ingredients just didn't exist before, and when these types of food products first came on the market, their flavor and texture was not always what we hoped. Nonfat cheese felt rubbery and reduced-fat mayonnaise just didn't taste good. Fortunately, times have changed! Food manufacturers have done a good job of bringing quality, flavorful reduced-fat, low-fat, and nonfat products to our local grocery stores (and not just the specialty stores, but also mainstream grocery chains). Low-calorie ingredients are easier than ever to find, come in a variety of brands, and are high in quality and flavor, thus making cutting back on calories and fat easier than ever!

Let's look at where the bulk of calories and fat are found in most recipes. There are the obvious ingredients—oil, butter, and sugar. But other ingredients can sneak up on you, turning an otherwise lean dish into an unwanted high-calorie one—ingredients such as whole milk, heavy whipping cream, rich buttermilk, traditional all-purpose flour, cream cheese, pesto sauces, traditional cream sauces, and mayonnaise, to name a few. A tablespoon here, ¼ cup there . . . calories and fat can add up fast and will translate to unwanted pounds. But with the help of this book, you can take control of the amount of calories in your recipes and maintain the delicious flavor you desire.

In order to be able to substitute lower-calorie, healthier ingredients in recipes you can enjoy every day, it's a good idea to keep certain items on hand in your kitchen. Here are a few common ingredients you can use to replace high-calorie or high-fat options:

Canned diced tomatoes

Cayenne pepper

Dijon mustard

Egg Beaters or other egg substitutes

Fresh lemons

Fresh oranges

Lean turkey bacon

continued

Lean turkey ham

Lean, 95 percent fat-free ground turkey

Lean, 95 to 98 percent fat-free ground beef

Light olive oil

Low-carb flour tortillas

Mild, medium, or hot salsa

Nonfat cottage cheese

Nonfat cream cheese

Nonfat evaporated milk

Nonfat mayonnaise

Nonfat milk

Nonfat or reduced-fat buttermilk

Nonfat powdered milk

Nonfat ricotta cheese or skim milk ricotta

Nonfat sour cream

Nonfat sweetened condensed milk

Nonfat vanilla yogurt (more flavorful than plain)

Reduced-fat cheeses such as Monterey jack, mozzarella, sharp Cheddar, and feta

Splenda or other sugar substitute

Sugar-free pudding mix such as chocolate, vanilla, or lemon

Tomato paste

Unsweetened applesauce

Whole-wheat flour

Whole-wheat pastas such as fettuccini, spaghetti, lasagna, and penne

Whole-wheat, whole-grain English muffins

Whole-wheat pita bread

Whole-wheat sandwich bread

Whole-wheat, low-carb tortillas

Even if you make a healthy dip, for example, you can still end up eating way too many calories through the chip you're using to eat the dip. Here are some snacking essentials to have on hand to avoid such calorie pitfalls: Melba rounds, pita crisps, Ak-mak crackers, saltine crackers, or substitute fresh cucumber slices for crackers!

Fresh herbs are a great way to enhance the flavor of recipes without adding calories. If you are fortunate enough to have a small garden, grow basil, rosemary, thyme, mint, and cilantro. Or keep small pots of these herbs in your windowsill.

Freeing yourself from "yo-yo" dieting is a liberating experience that will help you to enjoy life more. Now, with *Substitute Yourself Skinny*, you have the tools you need to achieve diet freedom. These easy-to-follow recipes are designed to help you break the yo-yo habit and enjoy your favorite foods without the guilt and fear of gaining weight and loss of flavor. Plus, I share easy "Skinny Secrets" you can implement to help you prevent overeating, which leads to weight gain. You'll also see a nutritional breakdown so you can see the healthy difference and big impact that substitutions make on these recipes and ultimately, in your life.

jumpstart-your-day breakfasts

apple-pear butter on crispy wheat toast

The apple-pear butter here is the perfect substitution for heavy-on-fat butter and tastes more delicious.

3 ripe Anjou pears, peeled, cored, and chopped
3 Golden Delicious apples, peeled, cored, and chopped
1¼ cups water
2 tablespoons fresh lemon juice
3 tablespoons honey
4 slices whole-wheat bread, toasted

Skinny Secret

Use this Apple-Pear Butter to add flavor to other dishes such as cooked chicken, pork chops, or even eggs!

In heavy saucepan over medium heat, combine all the ingredients, except the toast, and stir. Cover and simmer for 12 minutes, until the fruit begins to break down. Uncover and cook for an additional 5 to 7 minutes. Remove from heat and purée until smooth in food processor or blender. For a thinner mixture, add a little water. For a thicker mixture, add 1 teaspoon of cornstarch dissolved in 1 teaspoon of water. Spread on the toast. Refrigerate any remaining Apple-Pear Butter in an airtight container for up to 3 weeks.

SERVES 4	
Serving size	1 slice toast with 2 tablespoons Apple-Pear Butter

CALORIES PER SERVING	
Original recipe	110
SYS recipe	70

NUTRITIONAL BREAKDOWN	
Fat	1g
Carbohydrates	12g
Protein	1g
Sodium	132mg

mexicali low-cali breakfast burrito

The key substitution here is the low-fat whole-wheat tortillas. Not only is the whole wheat more easily digestible, 1 tortilla has only 2.5 grams of fat compared to 9 in regular tortillas.

¼ avocado, diced
Small squeeze of fresh lemon juice
Nonstick cooking spray
3 eggs, beaten
2 green onions, chopped
½ cup grated low-fat Monterey jack cheese
½ cup salsa
2 medium low-fat whole-wheat tortillas
½ cup nonfat sour cream (optional)

Toss the avocado with the lemon juice. Set aside. Spray a medium saucepan with nonstick cooking spray and heat over medium heat. Add the eggs and scramble until just cooked. Equally divide the eggs, onions, cheese, and salsa between the two tortillas and roll up to form a burrito. Top with sour cream if desired.

Skinny Secret

This recipe uses the whole egg. For an even leaner burrito, use only the egg whites—most of the fat and calories are in the yolk!

SERVES 2		CALORIES PER SERVING		NUTRITIONAL BREAKDOWN	
Serving size	1 burrito with sour cream	Original recipe	498	Fat	20g
		SYS recipe	406	Carbohydrates	29g
				Protein	18g
				Sodium	642mg

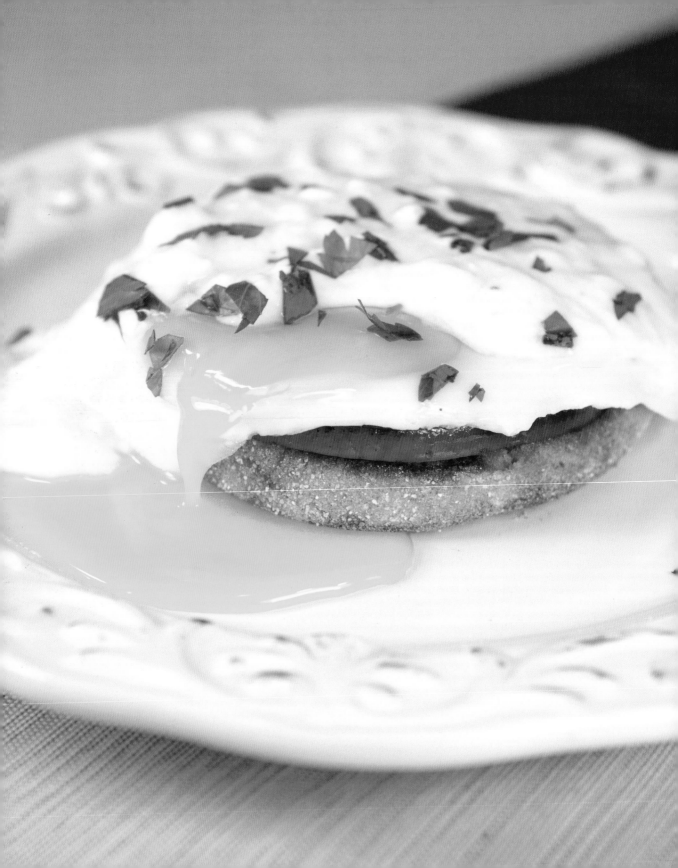

flat-belly eggs benedict

Get maximum flavor and creaminess by substituting nonfat vanilla yogurt, nonfat sour cream, and low-fat cottage cheese instead of butter and egg yolks. Turkey ham is also leaner than traditional deli ham.

2 multigrain English muffins

¼ cup nonfat vanilla yogurt

¼ cup nonfat sour cream

¼ cup low-fat cottage cheese

½ tablespoon fresh lemon juice

½ teaspoon Dijon mustard

¼ teaspoon sea salt

¼ teaspoon white pepper

4 tablespoons water

Nonstick cooking spray

4 eggs

3 slices deli sliced turkey ham, sliced into thirds

2 tablespoons chopped fresh Italian flat-leaf parsley

1. Preheat broiler. Toast the muffins in a toaster until golden. Set aside. In a small to medium mixing bowl, whisk together the yogurt, sour cream, cottage cheese, lemon juice, mustard, salt, and pepper. Set aside.

2. Spray a skillet with nonstick spray and heat on medium-low to medium. Add the water and heat until bubbling slightly. Add the eggs, whole; do not stir. Spoon the water over the eggs to cook the yolks slightly, about 1 minute. Transfer the eggs to a plate and set aside.

3. Place the English muffins on a baking tray, top each with approximately 2 strips turkey ham, then top with an egg, and spoon yogurt sauce on top. Top with parsley and place under the broiler for 30 seconds to 1 minute to heat sauce. Serve 1 muffin half per person.

Skinny Secret

If you nibble while you cook, you're eating extra calories fast with no way to keep track of them. To prevent nibbling while cooking, premix or precut the ingredients the day or night before, when you're full and less likely to snack. In this recipe, you could premix the yogurt mixture and slice the muffins the day before, so you are ready to cook immediately, therefore minimizing nibbling opportunities.

SERVES 4	
Serving size	½ muffin with 1 egg, ¾ slice ham, and 2 tablespoons sauce

CALORIES PER SERVING	
Original recipe	590
SYS recipe	179

NUTRITIONAL BREAKDOWN	
Fat	9.5g
Carbohydrates	16g
Protein	8.5g
Sodium	394mg

very veggie breakfast burrito

Low-carb tortillas and low-fat mozzarella cheese contribute to your calorie and fat savings here. With a calorie savings of 357 per serving, you can't go wrong with this high-energy breakfast!

1 tablespoon olive oil
¼ cup chopped white or yellow onion
½ cup chopped red bell pepper
2 Roma tomatoes, seeded and diced
2 (4-inch) asparagus spears with tips, chopped
3 eggs, beaten
1 tablespoon chopped fresh basil leaves
½ cup shredded low-fat mozzarella cheese
2 medium low-carb flour tortillas

Skinny Secret

Low-carb tortillas still give you the energy your body needs but in smaller doses, so there's no need to feel guilty about enjoying this delicious and nutritious burrito! For an even lower-cal burrito, use only the egg whites and save an additional 41 calories per serving!

In medium saucepan over medium heat, heat the oil. Add the onions and sauté until tender, about 2 minutes. Add the peppers, tomatoes, and asparagus. Sauté until tender, about 2 to 3 minutes. Transfer the veggies to a bowl, and set aside. Scramble the eggs until just cooked. Equally divide all the ingredients, including the basil and mozzarella, among the tortillas and fold each into a burrito.

SERVES 2	
Serving size	1 burrito

CALORIES PER SERVING	
Original recipe	660
SYS recipe	303

NUTRITIONAL BREAKDOWN	
Fat	20g
Carbohydrates	29g
Protein	18g
Sodium	642mg

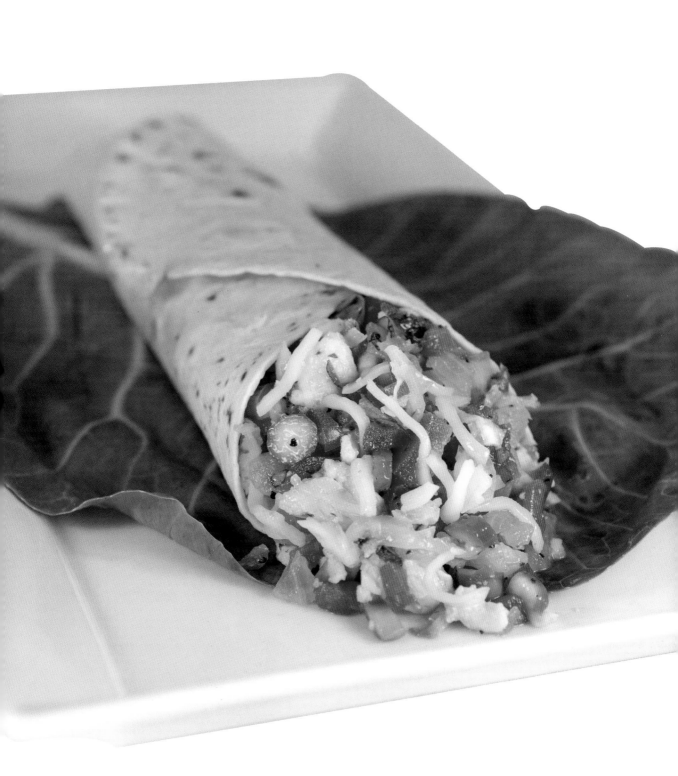

whole-wheat pancakes with raspberry syrup

Whole-wheat flour is a 100 percent whole-grain food and is therefore more nutritious than white flour. It's high in fiber and easily digestible, helping keep you lean. Due to its stronger wheat flavor, serve it with a low-fat sweet spread such as raspberry preserves.

2 cups whole-wheat flour
2 teaspoons baking powder
1 teaspoon sea salt
2 eggs, beaten
2 cups nonfat milk
2 tablespoons canola oil
Nonstick cooking spray
1 (13- to 16-ounce) jar sugar-free raspberry preserves
2 tablespoons water

Skinny Secret

Sugar-free preserves can be used on most anything and save you more than half the calories. Use them for sauces for chicken, pork, or for desserts!

1. Combine the flour, baking powder, and salt in a large bowl. In a separate bowl, combine the eggs, milk, and oil, and mix well. Pour into the dry ingredients and stir until just moistened.

2. Preheat a griddle to medium-high heat and spray with nonstick cooking spray. Pour about ¼ cup of the batter onto the griddle for each pancake. Cook until bubbles form in the center of pancake and the edges become dry. Using a flat spatula, flip the pancakes and cook until lightly browned.

3. In a small-quart boiler, heat the preserves with the water over medium heat. Stir until the mixture is warmed and slightly thin. Spoon 1 to 2 tablespoons of warm preserves over each pancake.

SERVES 8		CALORIES PER SERVING		NUTRITIONAL BREAKDOWN	
Serving size	2 pancakes with 2 table-spoons syrup	Original recipe	510	Fat	5g
		SYS recipe	173	Carbohydrates	36g
				Protein	5g
				Sodium	14mg

cinnamon-apple pancakes

Flavorful pancakes are often filled with sugar. Here, naturally sweet applesauce is used, giving a nice apple flavor and sweetness without processed sugar.

½ cup plain flour
1 teaspoon brown sugar
1 teaspoon baking powder
¼ teaspoon ground cinnamon
⅛ teaspoon sea salt
¼ cup nonfat milk
⅓ cup unsweetened applesauce
Nonstick cooking spray

1. In medium mixing bowl, combine the flour, sugar, baking powder, cinnamon, and salt. Mix well. Add the milk and applesauce, and stir to combine.

2. Heat a griddle to medium heat and spray with nonstick cooking spray. Pour about ¼ cup of batter onto the griddle for each pancake. Cook until the center begins to bubble and the edges are dry. Using a flat spatula, flip the pancakes and continue to cook until very lightly browned.

Skinny Secret

For a light syrup, drizzle with a tablespoon or two of honey.

SERVES 2	
Serving size	2 pancakes

CALORIES PER SERVING	
Original recipe	297
SYS recipe	77

NUTRITIONAL BREAKDOWN	
Fat	1g
Carbohydrates	18g
Protein	2g
Sodium	185mg

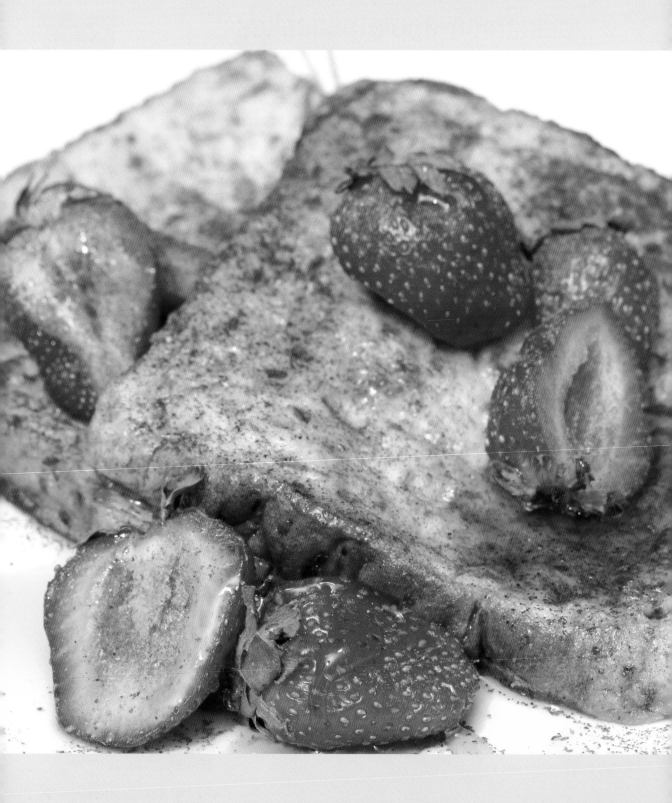

delectable french toast

CALORIE
SAVINGS
277

French toast is often made with large, thick slices of bread, which ratchets up the calorie and fat content. To satisfy your craving guilt-free, enjoy a smaller, lighter version and substitute egg whites for whole eggs and nonfat vanilla yogurt for whole milk in the batter.

½ cup nonfat vanilla yogurt
2 egg whites
½ pinch ground cinnamon
½ pinch ground nutmeg
4 slices "lite" Texas toast
Nonstick cooking spray

1. In medium mixing bowl, combine the yogurt, egg whites, cinnamon, and nutmeg. Dip the bread into the yogurt mixture, coating both sides.

2. Heat a griddle to medium heat. Spray with nonstick cooking spray. Place the toast on heated griddle and cook until browned on both sides, turning as needed. Serve the toast with 1 to 2 tablespoons sugar-free maple syrup and/or berries, if desired.

Skinny Secret

French toast can be very fattening. If you are at a restaurant enjoying the original version, share with a friend—or order something else!

SERVES 4	
Serving size	1 slice toast

CALORIES PER SERVING	
Original recipe	356
SYS recipe	79

NUTRITIONAL BREAKDOWN	
Fat	1g
Carbohydrates	95g
Protein	5g
Sodium	149mg

not-so french toast

Sweeten up your French toast with a little honey and fresh blueberries, which are high in antioxidants and natural sugars but low in calories.

2 egg whites
1 cup nonfat milk
Tiny pinch of cinnamon
1 tablespoon honey
2 slices whole-wheat bread
Nonstick cooking spray
¼ cup fresh blueberries

Skinny Secret

French toast is yummy on its own. Skip the extra-sugary syrup and substitute naturally sweet, healthy, fresh berries, as here.

1. In a medium mixing bowl, whisk together the egg whites, milk, cinnamon, and honey. Dip each slice of bread in the egg mixture, coating both sides.

2. Spray a griddle or skillet with nonstick spray and heat over medium heat. Place the prepared bread slices on the griddle and cook until browned on both sides. Remove from heat and serve with fresh blueberries.

SERVES 2	
Serving size	1 slice toast

CALORIES PER SERVING	
Original recipe	345
SYS recipe	161

NUTRITIONAL BREAKDOWN	
Fat	1g
Carbohydrates	27g
Protein	10g
Sodium	291mg

biscuits and gravy

Using the vegetarian sausage saves 144 calories per link!

For the biscuits:

1½ cups reduced-fat biscuit mix
½ cup nonfat milk

For the gravy:

½ pound vegetarian sausage, finely chopped
3 cups nonfat milk
¼ cup plain flour
⅛ teaspoon sea salt
¼ teaspoon ground black pepper

To make the biscuits:

1. Preheat oven to 450°F. Line a baking sheet with parchment paper or spray with nonstick spray. In a bowl, combine the biscuit mix and milk. Stir together until a soft dough forms. Turn out onto a lightly floured surface and roll into a circle about ½-inch thick using a lightly floured rolling pin. With a floured 2½-inch biscuit cutter, cut out 8 rounds.

2. Place the biscuits on the prepared baking sheet and bake for 8 to 10 minutes, or until lightly browned. Transfer the biscuits to a cooling rack.

To make the gravy:

1. In a large nonstick skillet, sauté the sausage over medium heat, breaking up any large lumps, for about 4 minutes. Transfer the sausage to a small bowl.

2. In medium bowl, whisk together the milk, flour, salt, and pepper just until the flour dissolves. Add the mixture to the same skillet and bring to a boil over medium heat, stirring frequently. Reduce heat and simmer, stirring frequently, for about 10 to 12 minutes or until thickened. Add the cooked sausage and heat for about 1 minute. Serve 2 tablespoons of gravy over 1 biscuit.

SERVES 8		CALORIES PER SERVING		NUTRITIONAL BREAKDOWN	
Serving size	1 biscuit with 2 tablespoons gravy	Original recipe	530	Fat	8g
		SYS recipe	273	Carbohydrates	36g
				Protein	14g
				Sodium	844mg

saucy sausage biscuits

Most of the fat in sausage biscuits and gravy is in full-fat sausage and whole milk. Substitute leaner turkey sausage and nonfat milk for significant calorie savings!

For the sausage biscuits:

1 recipe biscuit dough, see Biscuits and Gravy, page 13
8 turkey sausage patties

For the gravy:

3 cups nonfat milk
¼ cup plain flour
⅛ teaspoon sea salt
¼ teaspoon ground black pepper

Skinny Secret

It pays to shop around for calories! In this recipe alone, you save between 60 and 180 calories by substituting turkey sausage patties for pork sausage patties. However, even between brands, pork sausage patties can vary in calories and fat by as much as 200 percent.

1. Bake biscuits as directed in Biscuits and Gravy recipe, page 13.

2. Heat a medium skillet over medium heat. Add the sausage patties and cook until heated through, about 4 minutes. Remove from heat and wrap in aluminum foil to keep warm.

3. Prepare the gravy by whisking together the milk, flour, salt, and pepper in a medium bowl. Heat a medium skillet over medium heat and add the milk mixture. Bring to a boil, stirring often. Reduce heat and simmer, stirring occasionally, for about 15 minutes, until thickened. Slice the biscuits in half, place a sausage patty in between, and top each with 2 tablespoons of gravy.

SERVES 8		CALORIES PER SERVING		NUTRITIONAL BREAKDOWN	
Serving size	1 biscuit with 1 sausage patty	Original recipe	1,040	Fat	10g
		SYS recipe	278	Carbohydrates	84g
				Protein	14g
				Sodium	891mg

yummy waffles

Reduced-fat buttermilk is lower in fat and calories than regular buttermilk and whole milk. Combining natural oats and wheat flour keeps these waffles lighter in texture while packing in fiber, which aids in digestion.

2 cups reduced-fat buttermilk
½ cup quick-cooking oats
⅔ cup whole-wheat flour
⅔ cup plain flour
1½ teaspoons baking powder
½ teaspoon baking soda
¼ teaspoon sea salt
½ teaspoon ground cinnamon
2 egg whites, beaten
2 tablespoons light brown sugar
1 tablespoon canola oil
2 teaspoons vanilla extract
Nonstick cooking spray

Skinny Secret

Serve these healthy waffles with slices of fresh fruit such as peaches, bananas, or strawberries.

1. In medium mixing bowl, combine the buttermilk and oats. Let stand for 10 minutes. In another bowl, whisk together the wheat flour, plain flour, baking powder, baking soda, salt, and cinnamon.

2. In separate bowl, whisk together the eggs, sugar, oil, and vanilla. Add the dry ingredients to the wet ingredients and mix until just moistened.

3. Spray a waffle iron with nonstick spray. Using a ¼ cup measure, pour in enough batter to fill ⅔ of iron. Cook until lightly golden, about 4 minutes. Repeat with remaining batter. Serve warm.

SERVES 8		CALORIES PER SERVING		NUTRITIONAL BREAKDOWN	
Serving size	2 waffles	Original recipe	440	Fat	3g
		SYS recipe	154	Carbohydrates	25g
				Protein	7g
				Sodium	79mg

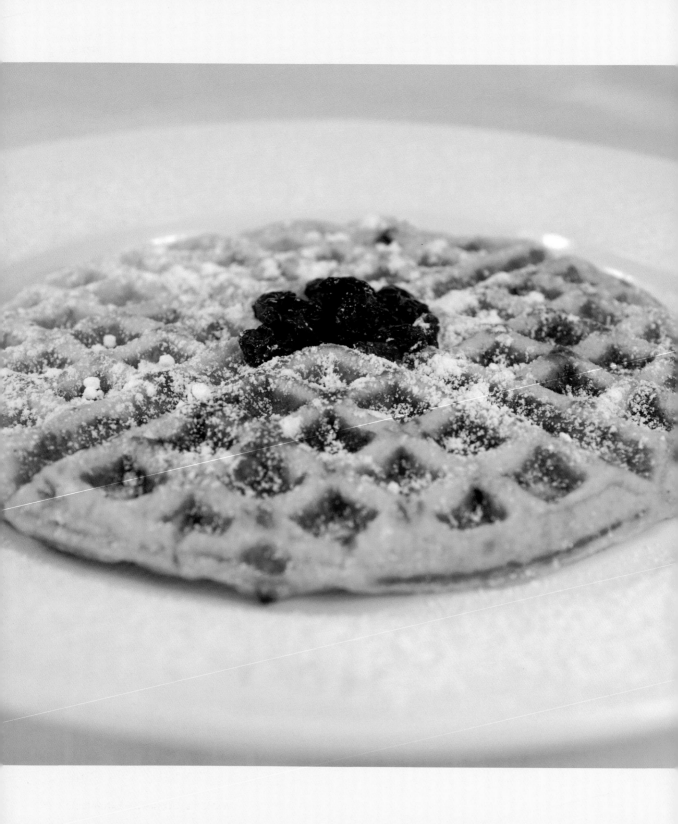

cinnamon raisin waffles

Key substitutions here are egg whites, reduced-fat buttermilk, and nonfat sour cream—all of which save on calories, fat, and even cholesterol!

2 cups plain flour

1½ tablespoons baking powder

½ teaspoon baking soda

3 tablespoons granulated sugar

½ teaspoon cinnamon

2 egg whites, beaten

2¼ cups reduced-fat buttermilk

¼ cup nonfat sour cream

1 teaspoon vanilla extract

½ cup raisins

Nonstick cooking spray

Skinny Secret

When waffles taste this good, it's easy to skip the syrup!

1. In a medium mixing bowl, combine the flour, baking powder, baking soda, sugar, and cinnamon. Mix well. In a separate mixing bowl, combine the egg whites, buttermilk, sour cream, vanilla, and raisins. Mix well.

2. Stir the dry ingredients into the wet ingredients just until combined. Spray a waffle iron with nonstick spray and heat to medium heat. Using a ¼ cup measure, pour batter into the waffle iron to fill ⅔ of the iron. Cook until lightly browned. Repeat with remaining batter and serve.

SERVES 8	
Serving size	1 waffle

CALORIES PER SERVING	
Original recipe	436
SYS recipe	189

NUTRITIONAL BREAKDOWN	
Fat	9g
Carbohydrates	39g
Protein	6g
Sodium	82mg

veggies never tasted so good omelet

Adding cottage cheese gives a more creamy texture to your omelet and adds a little extra protein while cutting calories! Substitute your favorite vegetables for these if you prefer.

Nonstick cooking spray
¼ cup chopped white onion
½ red bell pepper, chopped
¼ cup chopped fresh broccoli florets
3 eggs, beaten
1 tablespoon nonfat cottage cheese
1 pinch sea salt
1 pinch black pepper

1. Spray an omelet pan or medium sauté pan with nonstick spray and heat on medium. Add the onion, bell pepper, and broccoli, and sauté until just tender, about 4 minutes.

2. In medium mixing bowl, whisk together the eggs, cottage cheese, salt, and pepper. Pour half of the mixture into the omelet pan and cook until the bottom of the egg is very lightly golden. Add ½ the vegetable mixture to the center of the omelet, and gently fold one side of the omelet over the other. Cook for an additional 30 seconds to 1 minute. Remove from heat and serve. Repeat with remaining ingredients.

SERVES 2	
Serving size	1 omelet

CALORIES PER SERVING	
Original recipe	258
SYS recipe	91

NUTRITIONAL BREAKDOWN	
Fat	6g
Carbohydrates	1g
Protein	9g
Sodium	125mg

simply delish turkey omelet

CALORIE SAVINGS

281

Lean turkey, egg whites, and nonfat milk all help to reduce calories, fat, and cholesterol. As well, skipping the butter and using nonstick cooking spray is another great way to cut out unwanted calories.

Nonstick cooking spray

2 slices lean deli meat turkey, chopped

¼ cup chopped white or yellow onion

6 egg whites

2 tablespoons nonfat milk

1 pinch sea salt

1 pinch black pepper

1. Spray a medium saucepan with nonstick spray and heat on medium. Add the turkey and onion, and sauté until the onion is tender, about 3 minutes. Transfer the onion mixture to a small bowl and set aside.

2. Separately, whisk together the egg whites, milk, salt, and pepper. Pour half of the egg mixture into the pan. Cook for about 1 minute, until slightly firm. Add half the turkey mixture to center of the omelet. Gently fold one half of the omelet over the other half. Let cook for an additional minute. Remove from pan. Repeat with remaining ingredients and serve.

Skinny Secret

You can substitute extra-lean deli ham, if you prefer, as it is similar in calorie and fat content.

SERVES 2	
Serving size	1 omelet

CALORIES PER SERVING	
Original recipe	360
SYS recipe	79

NUTRITIONAL BREAKDOWN	
Fat	1g
Carbohydrates	15g
Protein	2g
Sodium	386mg

oh my eggs omelet

Substituting cheese made with 2% milk or reduced-fat cheese saves a whopping 65 calories per serving and over 7 grams of fat. Add to that the fat, calories, and cholesterol saved by using egg whites, and you've got significant savings. As well, adding a splash of calorie-free Sprite Zero or Sierra Mist Free makes for fluffy eggs without adding calories.

6 egg whites
Splash of Sprite Zero or Sierra Mist Free
1 pinch sea salt
1 pinch black pepper
Nonstick cooking spray
2½ tablespoons 2% milk Cheddar cheese

Skinny Secret

Egg whites are high in protein and potassium, giving you strength and aiding in muscle control.

1. In medium mixing bowl, whisk together the egg whites, Sprite or Sierra Mist, salt, and pepper.

2. Spray an omelet pan or medium skillet with nonstick spray and heat on medium. Pour in half of the egg mixture and cook for about 1 minute, until slightly firm. Add 1¼ tablespoons of cheese to the center of omelet. Gently fold half of the omelet over the other half. Allow to cook for an additional minute or until the egg is cooked through. Repeat with remaining ingredients and serve.

SERVES 2		CALORIES PER SERVING		NUTRITIONAL BREAKDOWN	
Serving size	1 omelet	Original recipe	132	Fat	1g
		SYS recipe	71	Carbohydrates	.9g
				Protein	14g
				Sodium	233mg

ginchy quiche

Most quiche recipes call for heavy whipping cream, which can really
pack on the pounds.

1 pinch sea salt, plus more to taste
3 cups broccoli florets
2 tablespoons olive oil
1 medium-sized yellow onion, chopped
1 clove fresh garlic, peeled and chopped
¼ teaspoon cayenne pepper
Black pepper to taste
1 (9-inch) pie crust
3 eggs, beaten
1 cup nonfat milk
1 cup nonfat sour cream

1. Preheat oven to 375°F. Fill a large-quart boiler halfway with water
and heat on medium-high. Add a pinch of sea salt. Bring the water to
a boil, and add the broccoli. Allow to boil for 30 seconds. Transfer the
broccoli to strainer and drain. Coarsely chop the larger florets, leaving
chunky bites of broccoli.

2. Heat the oil in large skillet over medium heat. Add the onion and
sauté until just tender, about 4 minutes. Add the broccoli, garlic, and
cayenne pepper. Season with salt and pepper to taste. Sauté for
about 3 to 4 minutes. Transfer to the pie crust.

3. Separately, whisk together the eggs, milk, and sour cream. Pour
over the broccoli mixture. Bake for 35 minutes or until a toothpick
inserted comes out clean.

SERVES 8		CALORIES PER SERVING		NUTRITIONAL BREAKDOWN	
Serving size	⅛ slice of quiche	Original recipe	248	Fat	8g
		SYS recipe	163	Carbohydrates	14g
				Protein	10g
				Sodium	178mg

spectacular spinach quiche

These days, good-quality reduced-fat and nonfat ingredients are easy to find and taste good compared to their higher-fat counterparts.

1 tablespoon olive oil

1 medium-sized white or yellow onion, chopped

4 cups fresh spinach leaves, stems trimmed, leaves washed, dried, and chopped

½ cup chopped cremini mushrooms (optional)

Juice of ½ lemon

4 eggs, beaten

¼ cup reduced-fat buttermilk

¾ cup nonfat milk

1 cup nonfat plain yogurt

Small pinch of ground nutmeg

Sea salt and black pepper to taste

1 (9-inch) pie crust

Skinny Secret

In addition to nonfat sour cream, nonfat yogurt is a great substitution for heavy whipping cream, saving you 78 grams of fat per recipe alone, not to mention all the other tasty substitutions!

1. Preheat oven to 375°F. In a medium saucepan, heat the oil on medium and add the onion. Sauté until tender, about 5 minutes. Add the chopped spinach, mushrooms, and lemon juice. Sauté until the spinach is wilted, about 5 minutes. Drain excess moisture in strainer, pressing lightly to remove liquid.

2. Separately, whisk together the eggs, buttermilk, milk, yogurt, nutmeg, salt, and pepper.

3. Transfer the spinach mixture to the pie crust, spreading evenly. Pour the egg mixture over the spinach. Tent with foil so foil is not touching top of quiche. Bake for 20 minutes. Remove foil and bake an additional 20 minutes, or until a toothpick inserted comes out clean. Slice and serve.

4. *Note:* If desired, transfer the premade pie crust to a decorative, ovenproof pie dish sprayed with nonstick cooking spray (transfer it before adding the spinach and egg mixture).

SERVES 8	
Serving size	⅛ slice of quiche, about ¾ cup

CALORIES PER SERVING	
Original recipe	253
SYS recipe	135

NUTRITIONAL BREAKDOWN	
Fat	7g
Carbohydrates	14g
Protein	12g
Sodium	167mg

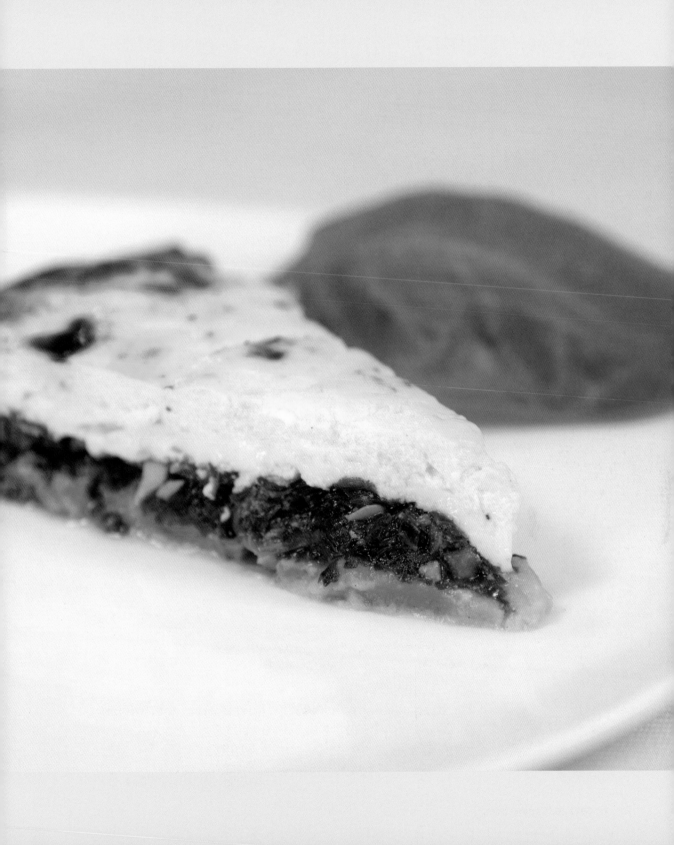

can't be quiche

Opportunities for substitutions in this recipe are practically endless. Lean turkey bacon, reduced-fat feta cheese, and nonfat milk and sour cream all work together to save calories while the fresh herbs maximize flavor.

4 slices lean turkey bacon
1 medium-sized white or yellow onion, chopped
5 eggs
½ cup reduced-fat feta cheese crumbles
½ tablespoon freshly chopped cilantro leaves
½ tablespoon freshly chopped Italian flat-leaf parsley leaves
1 cup nonfat milk
½ cup nonfat sour cream
Sea salt and black pepper to taste
1 (9-inch) pie crust

Skinny Secret

This quiche is so rich you can enjoy smaller slices, making it the skinniest of skinny quiche recipes.

1. Preheat oven to 375°F. In a medium skillet over medium heat, cook the bacon until crisp, about 5 minutes. Remove from heat and dice. Set aside. Wipe out half the grease from the skillet. Heat the remaining grease over medium heat and add the onion. Sauté until just tender, about 5 minutes. Set aside.

2. In a medium to large mixing bowl, whisk together the eggs, cheese, cilantro, parsley, milk, and sour cream, and season with salt and pepper. Whisk in the bacon and onion. Pour into the pie crust and tent with foil, making sure foil does not touch the top of the quiche. Bake for 20 minutes, then remove foil. Bake for an additional 15 to 20 minutes, or until a toothpick inserted comes out clean.

SERVES 10		CALORIES PER SERVING		NUTRITIONAL BREAKDOWN	
Serving size	⅒ slice of quiche	Original recipe	380	Fat	9g
		SYS recipe	147	Carbohydrates	10g
				Protein	12g
				Sodium	365mg

cheese blintzes

Cheese blintzes can be one of the most fattening breakfast foods. Save yourself the calories and guilt by using egg whites, nonfat milk, reduced-fat ricotta, low-fat cream cheese, a hint of sugar substitute, and applesauce for a deliciously skinny breakfast.

For the crepe batter:

¾ cup plain flour

1½ tablespoons granulated sugar

4 egg whites

¾ cup plus 3 tablespoons nonfat milk

½ teaspoon vanilla extract

1 pinch sea salt

1 tablespoon unsalted butter

For the cheese filling:

1½ cups reduced-fat ricotta cheese

4 ounces low-fat cream cheese, softened

1 egg white

1 tablespoon powdered sugar

1 tablespoon sugar substitute

Fine zest of 1 lemon

For the topping:

½ cup nonfat sour cream

1 tablespoon honey

1 tablespoon applesauce

Nonstick cooking spray

1 recipe Apple-Pear Butter (page 2)

Skinny Secret

This is the perfect recipe for a light brunch. Serve with a side of fresh berries and that's all you need!

1. Make the crepe batter: In a medium mixing bowl, whisk together all the batter ingredients to form a smooth, thin batter. Refrigerate for at least 1 hour.

continued

SERVES 8		CALORIES PER SERVING		NUTRITIONAL BREAKDOWN	
Serving size	2 blintzes with 1 tablespoon Apple-Pear Butter	Original recipe	689	Fat	6g
		SYS recipe	151	Carbohydrates	18g
				Protein	7g
				Sodium	115mg

cheese blintzes

continued

2. Make the filling: In a medium mixing bowl, stir together all the filling ingredients until smooth. Chill the filling in the refrigerator until ready to use.

3. Make the topping: In a small bowl, whisk together all the topping ingredients until well combined. Keep in the refrigerator until ready to use.

4. Preheat oven to 400°F. Make the crepes: Spray a medium skillet with nonstick spray and heat on medium-high. Using a ¼ cup measure, pour the batter into the pan, tilting the pan to coat evenly with batter. Cook until golden brown on the bottom and the top begins to appear dry, about 2 minutes. Using a flat spatula, carefully flip the crepe to brown the other side. Remove from heat, transfer to a plate, and loosely cover with foil. Repeat with the remaining batter.

5. Form the blintzes by spooning ¼ cup of filling along the bottom third of each crepe. Fold the edges over the filling, and roll to seal. Arrange the crepes in the bottom of a baking dish, trying to get them all in one layer. Bake the blintzes until the bottoms are golden brown and the filling is set.

6. To serve, place 2 blintzes on a plate. Top each with 1 tablespoon Apple-Pear Butter and 1 tablespoon of the sour cream mixture. Serve immediately.

apricot-orange muffins

Natural foods such as high-fiber, whole-wheat flour, fresh orange juice, and nonfat milk aid in digestion while saving fat and calories. Using egg whites helps keep a lighter muffin texture while at the same time saving on calories and cholesterol.

Nonstick cooking spray

1½ cups whole-wheat flour

¼ cup brown sugar

1 teaspoon baking powder

½ teaspoon baking soda

½ teaspoon sea salt

Fine zest of ½ an orange

½ cup fresh orange juice (not from concentrate)

½ cup nonfat milk

2 egg whites

½ cup chopped dried apricots

1. Preheat oven to 400°F. Spray muffin tins with nonstick spray. In a mixing bowl, combine the flour, sugar, baking powder, baking soda, and salt. Mix well. Separately, combine the orange zest, juice, milk, and egg whites. Mix well. Stir the orange mixture into the flour mixture until just combined. Fold in the apricots until blended.

2. Pour the batter into the prepared muffin cups and bake for 25 minutes or until a toothpick inserted comes out clean.

Skinny Secret

Often, Apricot-Orange Muffins are served with a powdered sugar glaze. Skip the glaze and drizzle ½ tablespoon of honey over them when serving for the natural sugar your body needs.

MAKES 12 MUFFINS	
Serving size	1 muffin

CALORIES PER SERVING	
Original recipe	238
SYS recipe	104

NUTRITIONAL BREAKDOWN	
Fat	1g
Carbohydrates	24g
Protein	3g
Sodium	16mg

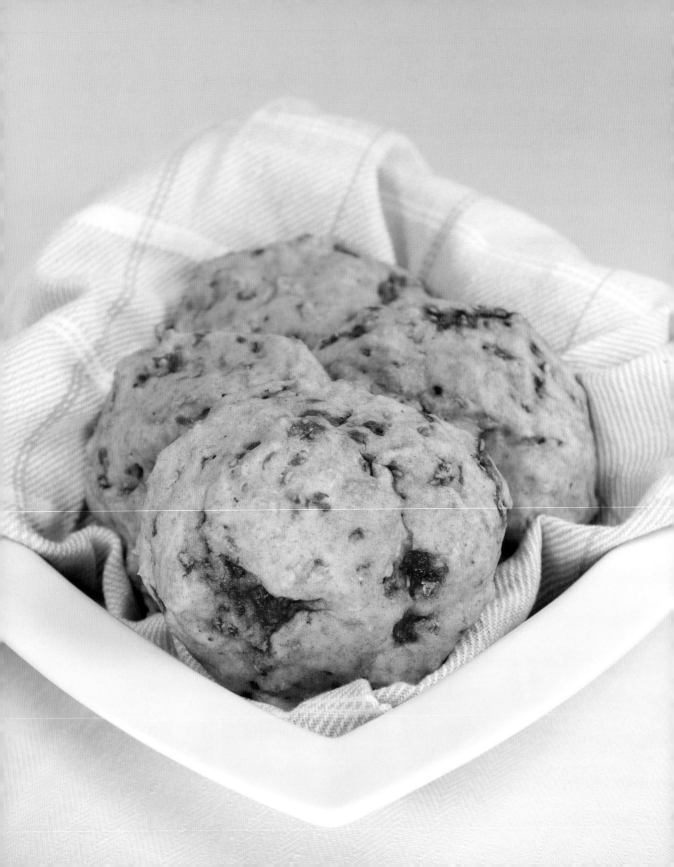

berry merry biscuits

Most biscuit recipes call for shortening, which is actually fat! Here you use a minimal amount of canola oil and a little water.

½ cup plain flour
½ cup whole-wheat flour
¼ cup rolled oats
2 tablespoons bran cereal
2 tablespoons granulated sugar
1 teaspoon baking powder
¼ teaspoon sea salt
⅓ cup nonfat milk
¼ cup water
3 tablespoons canola oil
⅓ cup fresh raspberries (or your preferred berry)

1. Preheat oven to 400°F. Line a baking sheet with parchment paper or spray with nonstick spray. In a medium bowl, combine the plain flour, wheat flour, oats, cereal, sugar, baking powder, and salt. Mix well.

2. Separately, combine the milk, water, and oil in a small mixing bowl. Mix well. Stir the milk mixture into the flour mixture until just combined. Fold in the berries.

3. In about ⅓ cup increments, spoon the batter onto prepared baking sheet, about 2 inches apart. Bake for 18 to 20 minutes or until lightly browned. Serve warm.

Skinny Secret

Food that looks amazing tastes amazing! Adding naturally low-cal, low-fat berries makes this usually bland biscuit not only pretty but also good for you.

SERVES 6		CALORIES PER SERVING		NUTRITIONAL BREAKDOWN	
Serving size	1 biscuit	Original recipe	354	Fat	7g
		SYS recipe	171	Carbohydrates	23g
				Protein	18g
				Sodium	29mg

ham it down breakfast casserole

Similar to a breakfast frittata, this casserole is perfect made ahead of time. Combining eggs and egg whites saves more than 100 calories.

Nonstick cooking spray
7 slices whole-wheat bread, crusts removed, cut into cubes
2 cups shredded reduced-fat Cheddar cheese
1¼ cups chopped turkey ham
½ white or yellow onion, chopped
¼ cup chopped red bell pepper
3 eggs, beaten
4 egg whites, beaten
3 cups nonfat milk
Sea salt and black pepper to taste

Skinny Secret

Just the word "casserole" often brings a visual of a high-fat, high-carb dish. This leaner version is high in protein and good carbs to give you energy all the way to lunch and beyond.

1. Spray a 12-inch casserole dish with nonstick spray and place the bread cubes in the bottom. Sprinkle with the cheese, turkey ham, onion, and bell pepper. Set aside. In a large mixing bowl, combine the eggs, egg whites, milk, and salt and pepper. Whisk together well and pour over the cheese mixture. Cover and refrigerate for 8 hours.

2. Preheat oven to 350°F. Remove casserole from refrigerator and let rest for 15 minutes. Bake uncovered for 40 minutes, or until set.

SERVES 10	
Serving size	¹⁄₁₀ slice of casserole

CALORIES PER SERVING	
Original recipe	452
SYS recipe	150

NUTRITIONAL BREAKDOWN	
Fat	6g
Carbohydrates	20g
Protein	14g
Sodium	455mg

energizing lunches

new-you england clam chowder

Turkey bacon is key to making this popular chowder leaner than traditional chowder.

1 slice turkey bacon, chopped

½ large white onion, diced

1¾ cups water

2 baking potatoes, peeled, largely cubed

1½ teaspoons sea salt

1 teaspoon freshly ground black pepper

1 cup nonfat sour cream

½ cup nonfat milk

1 (10-ounce) can minced clams, drained, liquid reserved

1 tablespoon cornstarch dissolved in 2 tablespoons water

1. In a large-quart boiler (not a saucepan!) over medium heat, cook the bacon and onion. Sauté until the bacon is cooked and the onion is softened, about 5 minutes. Add the water and potatoes, and season with salt and pepper. Bring to a boil and continue boiling until the potatoes are just tender, about 15 minutes. Whisk in the sour cream and milk. Simmer for 10 minutes.

2. Add the clams and half of the clam juice, then whisk in the cornstarch mixture. Allow to simmer for an additional 10 minutes. Serve in 1-cup portions as an entrée or ½-cup portions as a side dish or first course.

Skinny Secret

Serving yourself smaller portions more frequently helps keep your tummy feeling full without consuming extra unwanted calories. Measure soups with a measuring cup so you know exactly how much you are consuming and serve in smaller bowls or cups.

SERVES 4		CALORIES PER SERVING		NUTRITIONAL BREAKDOWN	
Serving size	1 cup	Original recipe	396	Fat	2g
		SYS recipe	250	Carbohydrates	29g
				Protein	12g
				Sodium	164mg

cheesy veggie soufflé

Substituting egg whites for even some of the eggs cuts out calories, fat, and cholesterol. As well, instead of coating your soufflé dish with butter, use nonfat cooking spray!

1 pound fresh asparagus, stems trimmed, cut into ½ inch pieces
3 tablespoons butter
3 tablespoons chopped green onions
2 tablespoons plain flour
¾ cup nonfat milk
½ cup shredded reduced-fat Swiss cheese
1 pinch sea salt
1 pinch black pepper
1 pinch nutmeg
Fine zest of 1 lemon
3 egg yolks, beaten
6 egg whites, stiffly beaten
Nonstick cooking spray

Skinny Secret

Asparagus is used here, but you can substitute broccoli or green beans if you prefer. Prepare the same way.

1. Spray a round 2-quart baking dish with nonstick spray. Fill a large-quart boiler ¾ of the way with water and add a pinch of sea salt. Bring to a boil over medium-high heat, add the asparagus, and boil for 30 seconds. Remove and drain. Reserve ¼ cup of liquid; discard the rest.

2. Preheat oven to 375°F. In a sauté pan, melt the butter over medium heat. Add the onions and sauté until just tender, about 4 minutes. Add the flour and stir until blended. Add the milk and asparagus liquid. Stir until thickened. Add the cheese, salt, pepper, nutmeg, and lemon zest. Stir until cheese is melted and mixture is thickened.

3. Add the beaten egg yolks to a medium mixing bowl. Whisk in ⅓ of the cheese mixture. Whisk well. Whisk in the remaining cheese mixture. Add the asparagus and mix well. Fold in the egg whites. Transfer to baking dish and bake for 30 to 35 minutes. Serve by slicing into 8 equal portions, using a thin spatula to remove the slices from the pan.

SERVES 8	
Serving size	⅛ slice of soufflé

CALORIES PER SERVING	
Original recipe	327
SYS recipe	127

NUTRITIONAL BREAKDOWN	
Fat	5g
Carbohydrates	17g
Protein	8g
Sodium	20mg

chicken tacos

Avocados are naturally high in fat. Although they have the "good" fats your body needs, cutting back on the amount used reduces both calories and fat but keeps the avocado flavor in. Lean chicken breasts, low-fat cheese, and low-carb tortillas are all great ways to find extra calorie savings here and there.

¾ cup shredded cooked boneless, skinless chicken breasts
1 (4-ounce) can green chilies
4 small low-carb soft corn tortillas
1½ cups shredded iceberg lettuce
½ cup shredded low-fat Monterey jack cheese
¼ cup prepared guacamole
½ cup chopped white or yellow onions
½ cup prepared salsa

Skinny Secret

There are a thousand ways to make tacos. Try to stick with low-fat cheeses in moderation, and use abundant amounts of freshly chopped vegetables. For added flavor without the calories, add a pinch of freshly chopped cilantro!

1. In medium saucepan over medium heat, warm the chicken with green chilies until just heated, about 4 minutes. Loosely wrap the tortillas in paper towels and heat in the microwave for 12 to 15 seconds.

2. To serve: Equally divide the chicken mixture among the tortillas. Top each with equal amounts lettuce, cheese, guacamole, onions, and salsa. Or, arrange as desired.

SERVES 4	
Serving size	1 taco

CALORIES PER SERVING	
Original recipe	285
SYS recipe	158

NUTRITIONAL BREAKDOWN	
Fat	13g
Carbohydrates	14g
Protein	22g
Sodium	729mg

tune-up tuna salad

Add lemon juice and a hint of curry powder to spruce up tuna salad without adding those unwanted calories!

1 (6-ounce) can tuna in water, drained
1 stalk celery, finely chopped
2 tablespoons nonfat mayonnaise
¼ teaspoon curry powder
2 teaspoons fresh lemon juice
¼ cup halved red or green grapes
2 tablespoons chopped yellow onion
Sea salt to taste
Black pepper to taste
4 red leaf lettuce leaves, washed and dried

In a medium mixing bowl, combine the tuna, celery, mayonnaise, curry powder, lemon juice, grapes, and onion. Mix well. Season with salt and pepper. Serve on the lettuce leaves.

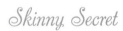

Skinny Secret

When using canned tuna, choose tuna in water as opposed to tuna in oil, which packs an additional 140 calories and a whopping 13 grams of fat per recipe.

SERVES 4	
Serving size	½ cup

CALORIES PER SERVING	
Original recipe	504
SYS recipe	57

NUTRITIONAL BREAKDOWN	
Fat	.4g
Carbohydrates	2g
Protein	11g
Sodium	182mg

lots o' flavor chicken salad on papaya boat

Substituting nonfat vanilla yogurt for high-fat mayonnaise not only reduces the calories and fat, but also adds a delicious element of flavor to this salad favorite. Omitting cooking oil and poaching the chicken in water is healthy and nearly fat-free.

Nonstick cooking spray
1 boneless, skinless chicken breast, chopped into 2-inch cubes
¼ cup water, or as needed
½ cup nonfat vanilla or plain yogurt
½ tablespoon honey
¼ teaspoon sea salt
¼ teaspoon freshly ground black pepper
1 teaspoon fresh finely grated lemon zest
½ cup green seedless grapes, halved
¼ cup chopped celery
2 papayas, halved and seeded

1. Spray a medium skillet with nonstick spray and heat on medium. Add the chicken and 2 tablespoons water. Cover and simmer for 5 minutes, adding water as needed to prevent burning. Cook the chicken until done, about 2 minutes longer. Remove from heat and set aside to cool.

2. In medium mixing bowl, combine the yogurt, honey, salt, pepper, and lemon zest, and whisk until well combined. Toss with the grapes, celery, and chicken until well coated. Spoon equally into the papaya halves.

Skinny Secret

Part of feeling satisfied when eating includes tantalizing your taste buds with a variety of textures and flavors. In this recipe, the creaminess of the yogurt mixture soothes the palate while your other taste buds enjoy the crunch of fresh celery and the heartiness of the chicken.

SERVES 4	
Serving size	½ papaya with ½ cup chicken salad

CALORIES PER SERVING	
Original recipe	220
SYS recipe	139

NUTRITIONAL BREAKDOWN	
Fat	<1g
Carbohydrates	18g
Protein	8g
Sodium	29mg

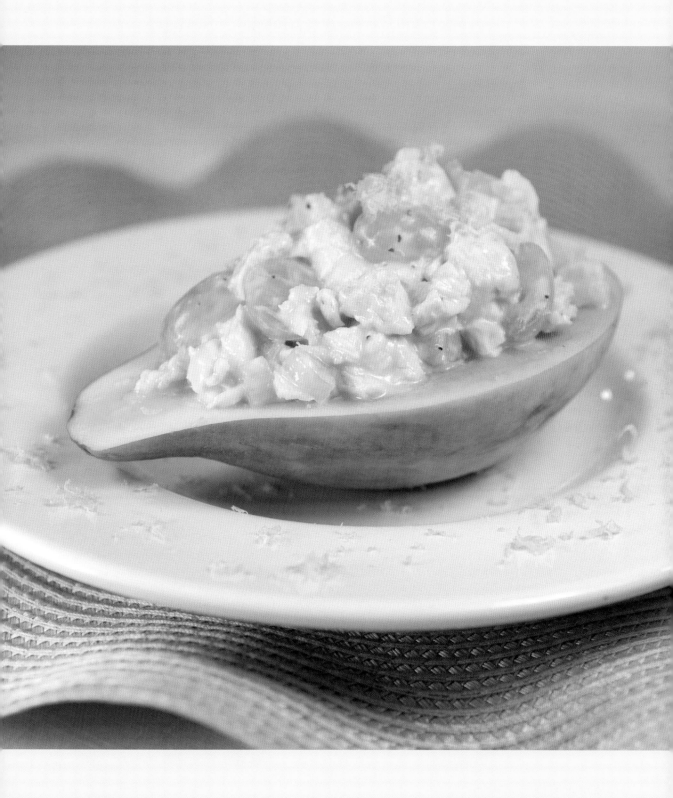

wow, that's a caesar salad

This Caesar salad dressing has so much flavor to it that you don't miss the overly fattening regular mayonnaise. Also, skipping on the croutons saves over 75 calories alone!

3 cloves garlic, minced

¾ cup nonfat mayonnaise

3 tablespoons grated Parmesan cheese

2 teaspoons Worcestershire sauce

1 teaspoon Dijon mustard

1 tablespoon fresh lemon juice

Sea salt to taste

Black pepper to taste

1 head romaine lettuce, washed, dried, and chopped into
    2-inch pieces

1. In large mixing bowl, whisk together the garlic, mayonnaise, cheese, Worcestershire, mustard, and lemon juice. Season to taste with salt and pepper. Toss with the lettuce to coat.

2. Serve on salad or dinner plates as an entrée or side dish.

Skinny Secret

One of the key flavors of this recipe is Dijon mustard, which is very bikini-friendly. Use Dijon mustard in marinades for chicken, pork, beef, and even vegetables.

SERVES 6	
Serving size	⅙ recipe, or 1 heaping cup

CALORIES PER SERVING	
Original recipe	384
SYS recipe	51

NUTRITIONAL BREAKDOWN	
Fat	1g
Carbohydrates	15g
Protein	2g
Sodium	282mg

shrimp louie salad

Shrimp Louie salad is usually made with heavy whipping cream, which lives up to its name—it's heavy in fat and high in calories. Substituting nonfat sour cream keeps fat and calories to a minimum, and the lemon juice kicks up the flavor!

½ cup chopped green onions

¼ cup chili sauce

1 teaspoon chopped fresh Italian flat-leaf parsley leaves

¼ teaspoon cayenne pepper

¼ cup nonfat sour cream

Juice of ½ lemon

1 head iceberg lettuce, shredded

1 pound cooked bay shrimp, peeled and deveined

2 tomatoes, quartered

2 hard-boiled eggs, sliced

1. In a large mixing bowl, combine the onions, chili sauce, parsley, cayenne pepper, sour cream, and lemon juice. Mix well.

2. Place the shredded lettuce in serving bowls. Layer with shrimp, arrange 2 tomato wedges in each bowl, and top with egg slices and approximately 2 tablespoons of sauce. Serve chilled.

Skinny Secret

Fresh, crisp, green onions are a nifty little way to add an edgy crunch to salads and all kinds of recipes. And, best of all, they're the ultimate in skinny!

SERVES 4		CALORIES PER SERVING		NUTRITIONAL BREAKDOWN	
Serving size	½ cup	Original recipe	581	Fat	5g
		SYS recipe	199	Carbohydrates	12g
				Protein	33g
				Sodium	334mg

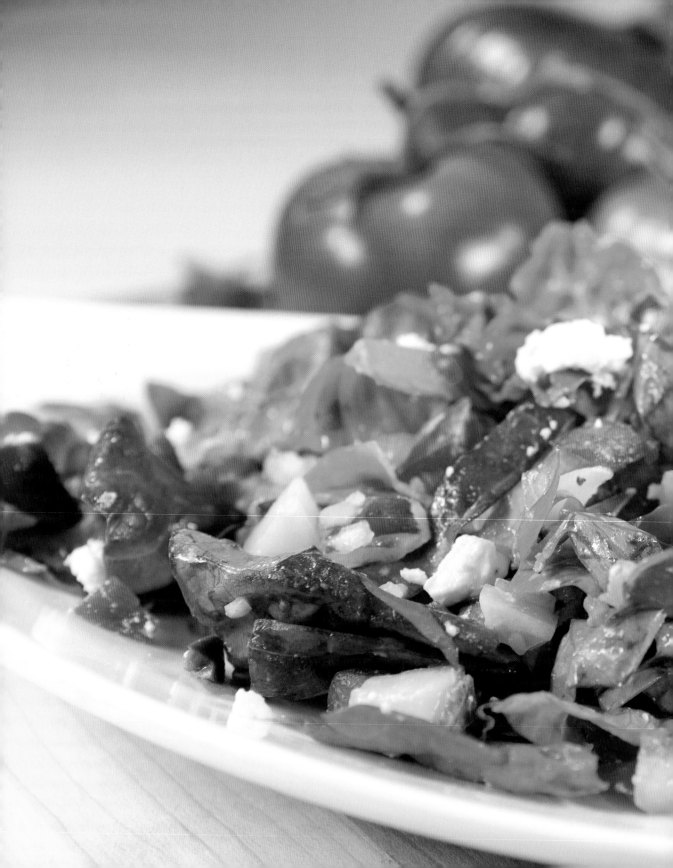

it's greek to me greek salad

Substitutions such as reduced-fat or nonfat feta cheese save on calories and fat; however, cutting back on the amount of extra-virgin olive oil in dressings is another key factor in keeping your recipes slimming.

½ head red leaf lettuce, washed, dried, and cut into
   2-inch pieces

1 English cucumber, diced

2 large tomatoes, diced

¼ cup chopped red onion

¼ cup chopped red bell pepper

¼ cup chopped pitted kalamata olives

½ cup reduced-fat feta cheese crumbles

1 teaspoon chopped fresh oregano leaves

2 tablespoons extra-virgin olive oil

2 teaspoons fresh lemon juice

Sea salt to taste

Black pepper to taste

1. In a large mixing bowl, toss together the lettuce, cucumber, tomatoes, onion, bell pepper, olives, and cheese. Separately, in small bowl, whisk together the oregano, oil, lemon juice, salt, and pepper. Pour over the lettuce mixture and toss well to coat.

2. Serve on salad plates as an entrée or side dish.

Skinny Secret

This recipe has so many great flavors in it that you can skip on the heavy salad dressing, which can add up to over 500 calories to an otherwise light salad.

SERVES 4	
Serving size	¾ cup

CALORIES PER SERVING	
Original recipe	440
SYS recipe	177

NUTRITIONAL BREAKDOWN	
Fat	15g
Carbohydrates	8g
Protein	4g
Sodium	469mg

spicy chinese noodles

Similar salads use a combination of mayonnaise and heavy cream. Skip on the cream to save on fat and calories. If you must have more creaminess, substitute ¼ cup of nonfat sour cream for ¼ cup of the mayonnaise.

1 head napa cabbage, shredded

1 cup chopped celery

1 bunch green onions, chopped

1 pound medium frozen shrimp, rinsed in cold water, drained

½ cup frozen green peas

1 cup Chinese noodles

1 cup nonfat mayonnaise

Juice of ½ lemon

¼ teaspoon Jane's Krazy Mixed-Up Salt (or other salt-spice blend of your choice)

Skinny Secret

Cutting back a little here and there can add up to significant savings. Lighten this dish even more by using only ¾ cup nonfat mayonnaise and save another 9 calories per serving.

In a mixing bowl, combine the lettuce, celery, and onions. Chill in the refrigerator for 30 minutes. When ready to serve, add the shrimp, peas, and noodles. Toss to combine. Add the mayonnaise, lemon juice, and salt, and toss to coat.

SERVES 4		CALORIES PER SERVING		NUTRITIONAL BREAKDOWN	
Serving size	½ cup	Original recipe	420	Fat	4g
		SYS recipe	285	Carbohydrates	34g
				Protein	30g
				Sodium	967mg

no-added-pad thai noodles

Many pad thai recipes are heavy on oil and sugar. Cutting back on the fat and adding in egg whites helps to keep this recipe lean.

8 ounces rice noodles

¼ cup low-sodium fish sauce

2 tablespoons brown sugar

2½ tablespoons low-sodium soy sauce

Juice of 1 lime

1 tablespoon rice wine vinegar

½ teaspoon cayenne pepper

1 tablespoon sesame oil

½ pound diced chicken breast

4 ounces firm tofu, cubed

3 cloves garlic, minced

1 egg, beaten

2 egg whites, lightly beaten

3 cup bean sprouts

4 medium green onions, chopped

2 tablespoons roughly chopped roasted, unsalted peanuts

½ tablespoon fresh lemon juice

¾ cup chopped fresh cilantro leaves

1. Bring a large pot of water to a boil. Remove from heat and add the noodles. Set aside while you prepare the other ingredients.

2. In medium mixing bowl, whisk together the fish sauce, sugar, soy sauce, lime juice, vinegar, cayenne pepper, and 1 teaspoon of the sesame oil. Set aside.

3. In medium saucepan over medium heat, heat the remaining sesame oil and add the chicken. Sauté until cooked through, about 3 minutes.

4. Add tofu and cook until browned, about 3 minutes. Add the garlic and cook for an additional 1 minute. Add the eggs and stir to combine. Add the chicken and sprouts. Cook until heated through, about 5 minutes. Stir in the drained noodles, green onions, and fish sauce mixture. Simmer until the mixture thickens, about 7 minutes.

5. To serve, place on plates and garnish with peanuts and cilantro.

SERVES 4		CALORIES PER SERVING		NUTRITIONAL BREAKDOWN	
Serving size	½ cup	Original recipe	700	Fat	11g
		SYS recipe	466	Carbohydrates	64g
				Protein	28g
				Sodium	561mg

chilly today hot tamale pie

Substituting lean turkey for higher-fat beef, egg whites for whole eggs, and nonstick cooking spray for cooking oil are all simple, easy ways to cut back on calories in everyday meals.

Nonstick cooking spray

1 tablespoon olive oil

1 white or yellow onion, chopped

1 red bell pepper, diced

¾ pound ground lean turkey

1 (15-ounce) can diced tomatoes

1 (12-ounce) can kernel corn (not cream style)

2 teaspoons chili powder

Sea salt to taste

Black pepper to taste

3 cups water

1 cup yellow cornmeal (or polenta)

2 egg whites, lightly beaten

Skinny Secret

This recipe also makes for a great, low-calorie appetizer. Simply spray a baking sheet with nonstick spray, spread the entire cornmeal mixture onto the baking sheet, top with an even coating of filling, and bake for about 20 minutes. Cut into squares and serve.

1. Preheat oven to 400°F. Spray a 2-quart oven-safe casserole dish with nonstick spray. In a large sauté pan, heat the oil on medium. Add the onion, bell pepper, and ground turkey. Sauté until the turkey is browned, about 5 minutes. Add the tomatoes, corn, and chili powder. Stir to combine. Season lightly with salt and pepper. Reduce heat, cover, and let simmer for about 5 minutes.

2. Meanwhile, bring 3 cups of water to boil in a small-quart boiler. When boiling, slowly stir in the cornmeal and continue stirring until very thick, about 5 to 6 minutes. Remove from heat and quickly stir in the eggs and a pinch of salt and pepper.

3. Spread ½ of the cornmeal mixture on the bottom of the casserole dish. Top with turkey filling. Spoon the remaining cornmeal mixture on top of the filling. Bake for 25 minutes or until nicely browned.

SERVES 12		CALORIES PER SERVING		NUTRITIONAL BREAKDOWN	
Serving size	¹⁄₁₂ of pie, about ½ cup	Original recipe	314	Fat	5g
		SYS recipe	157	Carbohydrates	17g
				Protein	11g
				Sodium	166mg

chinese chicken salad

Adding rice to salad makes for a filling recipe that is still low in calories. For an even more nutritious alternative, use brown rice, which is higher in fiber and protein.

½ cup nonfat plain yogurt
¼ teaspoon curry powder
¼ teaspoon chopped fresh gingerroot
1 teaspoon minced fresh garlic
Juice of ½ lemon
1½ cups cooked shredded chicken breasts
2 green onions, chopped
¼ teaspoon chili powder
1 pinch sea salt
1 tomato, diced
2 cups cooked white rice

1. In large a mixing bowl, combine the yogurt, curry powder, ginger, garlic, and lemon. Mix well and refrigerate for about 6 hours, stirring occasionally.

2. When ready to serve, add the chicken, onions, chili powder, salt, and tomato. Serve over ½ cup cooked rice.

Skinny Secret

Another low-cal addition to this salad is coarsely chopped water chestnuts. One-half cup is all you need and it adds only 15 calories per serving.

SERVES 4	
Serving size	½ cup

CALORIES PER SERVING	
Original recipe	455
SYS recipe	240

NUTRITIONAL BREAKDOWN	
Fat	1g
Carbohydrates	32g
Protein	24g
Sodium	82mg

melt-in-your-mouth tuna melt

For lighter recipes, always use canned tuna packed in water as opposed to oil. Also, substituting nonfat mayonnaise, reduced-calorie Italian dressing, and reduced-fat Monterey jack cheese all work together to keep fat and calories as low as possible while still maintaining the flavor and texture you love.

12 ounces canned light tuna in water, drained
1 shallot, finely chopped
2 tablespoons nonfat mayonnaise
Juice of ½ lemon
1 tablespoon chopped Italian flat-leaf parsley
1 dash hot sauce
1 tablespoon reduced-calorie Italian dressing
1 pinch sea salt
Black pepper to taste
8 slices whole-wheat bread, toasted
2 tomatoes, sliced
4 slices reduced-fat Monterey jack cheese

Skinny Secret

Save even more calories by skipping the additional piece of toast on top.

1. Preheat broiler. Line a baking sheet with parchment paper or spray with nonstick cooking spray. In a medium mixing bowl, combine the tuna, shallot, mayonnaise, lemon juice, parsley, hot sauce, dressing, salt, and pepper. Mix well. Place 4 slices of the toast on the prepared baking sheet. Top each with ¼ cup of tuna mixture, 1 tomato slice, and 1 slice of cheese.

2. Broil until the cheese is melted. Top with the additional piece of toast and serve.

SERVES 4	
Serving size	1 "melt"

CALORIES PER SERVING	
Original recipe	919
SYS recipe	334

NUTRITIONAL BREAKDOWN	
Fat	8g
Carbohydrates	43g
Protein	33g
Sodium	578mg

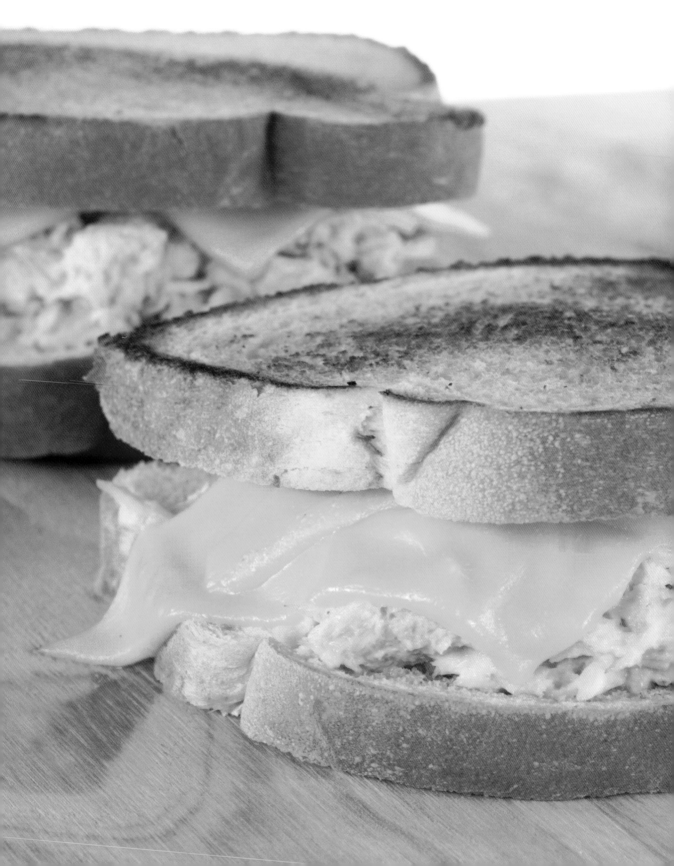

cheesiest cheese burrito

Reduced-fat whole-wheat tortillas are high in fiber and low in fat. Combined with reduced-fat cheeses and naturally low-in-fat enchilada sauce, you can enjoy your burrito guilt-free.

2 cups shredded lettuce
3 tomatoes, seeded and diced
3 tablespoons enchilada sauce
4 (8-inch) reduced-fat whole-wheat tortillas
1 cup shredded reduced-fat pepper jack cheese
1 cup shredded reduced-fat Cheddar cheese

1. In a small mixing bowl, combine the lettuce, tomatoes, and sauce. Mix well.

2. Lay 1 tortilla on a flat surface. Spread ¼ cup jack cheese and ¼ cup Cheddar cheese in the center of the tortilla. Top with ¼ cup of the lettuce mixture. Roll up the tortilla to form a burrito and enjoy.

Skinny Secret

Another alternative to this burrito recipe is to top the finished burrito with 1 tablespoon of additional cheese and place under the broiler to melt the cheese. This adds an additional 25 calories and 2 fat grams, but it is still less than the original recipe!

SERVES 4	
Serving size	1 burrito

CALORIES PER SERVING	
Original recipe	450
SYS recipe	265

NUTRITIONAL BREAKDOWN	
Fat	9g
Carbohydrates	39g
Protein	13g
Sodium	677mg

beef lovers' burrito

This recipe proves that beef burritos don't have to be fattening.
Use 80 to 95 percent lean ground beef and these other healthy
substitutions to cut calories but maintain the flavors and textures.

¾ pound lean ground beef

½ yellow or white onion, chopped

1 clove garlic, chopped

2 teaspoons chili powder

1 teaspoon chopped fresh oregano leaves

Sea salt to taste

Black pepper to taste

1 (10-ounce) can enchilada sauce

6 (8-inch) reduced-fat whole-wheat tortillas

2 cups shredded iceberg lettuce

Suggested toppings:

¾ cup fat-free refried beans

3 Roma tomatoes, seeded and chopped

½ cup nonfat sour cream

6 tablespoons shredded reduced-fat Cheddar cheese

1. In large skillet over medium heat, cook the ground beef, onion,
and garlic until the beef is browned, breaking up any large lumps.
Drain off the grease, and return the skillet to the stovetop. Add the
chili powder, oregano, salt, and pepper. Mix to combine, and sauté
for about 5 minutes. Add the enchilada sauce and stir to combine.
Simmer over low heat for about 8 minutes.

2. Wrap the tortillas loosely in paper towels and microwave for
15 seconds on high heat. Place 1 tortilla on a serving plate and
spread 2 tablespoons of refried beans on top. Top with ¼ cup of
the beef mixture, ⅓ cup of lettuce, and 1½ tablespoons each of
tomatoes, sour cream, and Cheddar cheese, if desired. Roll up the
tortilla to make a burrito. Repeat for remaining tortillas.

Skinny Secret

Adding your favorite toppings are part of what makes burritos so fun to make; however, remember fat and calories add up in the smallest of places. If you love sour cream, then skip the guacamole. If you can live without the cheese, skip it all together and save those calories for dessert!

SERVES 6	
Serving size	1 burrito

CALORIES PER SERVING	
Original recipe	450
SYS recipe	371

NUTRITIONAL BREAKDOWN	
Fat	12g
Carbohydrates	38g
Protein	28g
Sodium	1,059mg

deviled egg salad

Delicious salads don't need tons of mayonnaise. Use a reduced amount of mayonnaise and substitute nonfat mayonnaise for true calorie savings, and enjoy great flavor with naturally low-fat fresh dill, immune-boosting garlic, lemon, cayenne, and other delicious natural ingredients.

6 hard-boiled eggs
2 tablespoons nonfat mayonnaise
½ tablespoon chopped fresh dill
1 clove garlic, finely chopped
Fine zest of ½ lemon
½ teaspoon cayenne pepper
1 medium-sized dill pickle, chopped
½ teaspoon prepared mustard
¼ cup finely chopped red onion
Sea salt to taste
Black pepper to taste
1 head Boston leaf lettuce, washed and dried
½ cup grape tomatoes, left whole

Skinny Secret

The egg salad mixture can be made ahead of time and chilled before serving.

1. Gently peel the eggs, and carefully slice them in half, lengthwise. Carefully spoon out the yolks and transfer them to a large mixing bowl. Add the mayonnaise, dill, garlic, zest, cayenne, pickle, mustard, and onion. Mix well and season to taste with salt and pepper. Spoon about 1 tablespoon of egg yolk mixture into each egg half.

2. Arrange the lettuce leaves on serving plates and add 2 filled egg halves. Divide the tomatoes equally among the salads. Serve.

SERVES 4	
Serving size	½ cup

CALORIES PER SERVING	
Original recipe	269
SYS recipe	94

NUTRITIONAL BREAKDOWN	
Fat	6g
Carbohydrates	5g
Protein	9g
Sodium	364mg

niçoise salad

Most of the calories in a niçoise salad are in the vinaigrette, eggs, and olives. Making a light vinaigrette, as here, helps keep flavor in and calories out.

For the vinaigrette:

⅓ cup extra-virgin olive oil
⅓ cup champagne vinegar
1 teaspoon Dijon mustard
1 tablespoon chopped shallots
1 teaspoon dried Italian seasoning
Juice of ½ lemon
1 pinch sea salt
1 pinch black pepper

For the salad:

2 medium-sized new potatoes, cut into eighths
1 pinch salt
⅓ pound fresh green beans, rinsed and trimmed
4 cups mixed salad greens, washed and dried
¼ cup chopped fresh Italian flat-leaf parsley
1 (6-ounce) can light tuna in water, drained
¼ cup pitted niçoise olives
½ red onion, chopped
2 hard-boiled eggs, sliced
2 Roma tomatoes, seeded and chopped
1 tablespoon capers, drained

1. In medium mixing bowl, whisk together all the vinaigrette ingredients. Whisk until the oil thickens slightly. Set aside.

2. Fill a medium-quart boiler halfway with water. Bring to a boil over medium-high heat and add the potatoes. Cook until just fork-tender. (Do not overcook, as they will become mushy.) Fill a separate boiler halfway with water, add a pinch of salt, and bring to a boil. Add the beans and cook for 30 seconds. Using a slotted spoon, remove the beans and set aside to cool.

3. In a large salad bowl, toss the greens with the vinaigrette. Divide the salad among 4 plates. Top each with ¼ of the tuna, olives, onion, eggs, tomatoes, and capers. Serve.

SERVES 4	
Serving size	1 cup

CALORIES PER SERVING	
Original recipe	520
SYS recipe	110

NUTRITIONAL BREAKDOWN	
Fat	13g
Carbohydrates	14g
Protein	6g
Sodium	380mg

i'm not stuffed tomato salad

Substitute nonfat mayonnaise and add high-flavor Parmesan cheese, spices, and citrus to enjoy a delicious salad with minimal calories.

6 medium-sized ripe tomatoes
¼ cup diced red bell pepper
¼ cup seeded and diced cucumber
¼ cup diced red onion
1 (10-ounce) can kernel corn, drained
2 tablespoons grated Parmesan cheese
¼ cup nonfat mayonnaise
1 pinch cayenne pepper
Juice of ½ lemon
Sea salt to taste
Black pepper to taste

Skinny Secret

This simple salad is delicious as-is or with chopped cooked bay shrimp, which adds only 33 calories per 1-ounce serving and is more than enough for 1 tomato.

1. Place the tomatoes stem side down onto a cutting board. Cut each into 4 to 6 wedges, cutting just to but not through to the stem end. Cover and chill.

2. In a medium mixing bowl, combine the bell pepper, cucumber, onion, and corn. Toss to mix. Separately, in small bowl, mix together the Parmesan cheese, mayonnaise, cayenne, and lemon. Mix well and then pour over the vegetable mixture. Toss to coat well. Season with salt and pepper as desired. Spoon the salad mixture into the prepared tomatoes and serve.

SERVES 6	
Serving size	1 tomato with ½ cup salad

CALORIES PER SERVING	
Original recipe	196
SYS recipe	85

NUTRITIONAL BREAKDOWN	
Fat	2g
Carbohydrates	17g
Protein	4g
Sodium	208mg

lobster bisque

A dinner party favorite, the flavor in this dish is all about the lobster. Why ruin it with fat-laden heavy cream when you can substitute nonfat sour cream and maintain a creamy texture?

¼ cup apple cider vinegar

1 bay leaf

1 (1.5-pound) live lobster

1 tablespoon butter

1 shallot, finely chopped

½ carrot, peeled and largely chopped

2 tablespoons brandy

½ cup fish stock

3½ cups reserved lobster liquid

1 cup dry white wine such as sauvignon blanc

1 tablespoon chopped fresh tarragon

¾ cup nonfat sour cream

Juice of ½ lemon

1 pinch cayenne pepper

Sea salt to taste

Black pepper to taste

1. Fill a large-quart boiler ¾ of the way with water. Add the vinegar and bay leaf. Bring to a boil. Add the live lobster and cook for about 1 minute. Reduce heat to a simmer and let the lobster rest in the water an additional 4 minutes. Remove from heat. Remove the lobster and reserve the liquid. Allow the lobster to cool about 4 minutes. Crack the claws and remove the meat. Pull back the end of the tail to crack it and remove meat. Reserve the shells.

2. In another large-quart boiler over medium heat, melt the butter. Add the shallots and carrots; sauté for about 5 minutes. Add the brandy, fish stock, reserved liquid, and wine. Bring to a low boil and allow to boil for about 5 minutes. Add the tarragon and reserved lobster shells (the larger pieces) and reduce heat to a simmer. Simmer for 20 minutes. Add an additional ½ cup of reserved liquid if needed.

3. Remove the lobster shells from the liquid. Whisk in the sour cream, lemon, and cayenne. Season with salt and pepper as desired.

4. Chop the lobster into large bite-sized chunks and add half of the lobster to the soup. Working in batches, purée the soup in a food processor until smooth. Once puréed, return to the boiler and heat over low heat, stirring occasionally. When heated through, serve immediately with the remaining lobster pieces as garnish in the center of the serving dish.

SERVES 6		CALORIES PER SERVING		NUTRITIONAL BREAKDOWN	
Serving size	1 cup	Original recipe	251	Fat	3g
		SYS recipe	200	Carbohydrates	9g
				Protein	25g
				Sodium	544mg

i say tomato, you say tomoto bisque

Heavy cream is what the original version of this recipe is all about. Skip the cream without missing the creaminess by substituting a little nonfat sour cream and 1 potato. This delicious soup can be served hot or cold.

1 pound tomatoes, cut into eighths
2 cups low-sodium chicken broth
1 large new potato, cut into eighths
⅓ cup nonfat milk
⅓ cup nonfat sour cream
1 pinch cayenne pepper
Sea salt to taste
Black pepper to taste

1. In a large-quart boiler over medium heat, combine the tomatoes, broth, and potato. Bring to a low boil and let cook for 10 minutes or until the potato is tender. Add an additional ¼ cup of broth if needed. Reduce heat to a simmer and whisk in the milk, sour cream, and cayenne pepper. Season with salt and pepper to taste.

2. Working in batches, purée the soup in a food processor until smooth. Serve immediately.

Skinny Secret

Use this light, flavorful bisque as a base for other slimming soups by adding cooked fresh vegetables for tomato vegetable soup, or cooked bay scallops or shrimp for a seafood bisque.

SERVES 4		CALORIES PER SERVING		NUTRITIONAL BREAKDOWN	
Serving size	1 cup	Original recipe	253	Fat	1g
		SYS recipe	82	Carbohydrates	17g
				Protein	5g
				Sodium	637mg

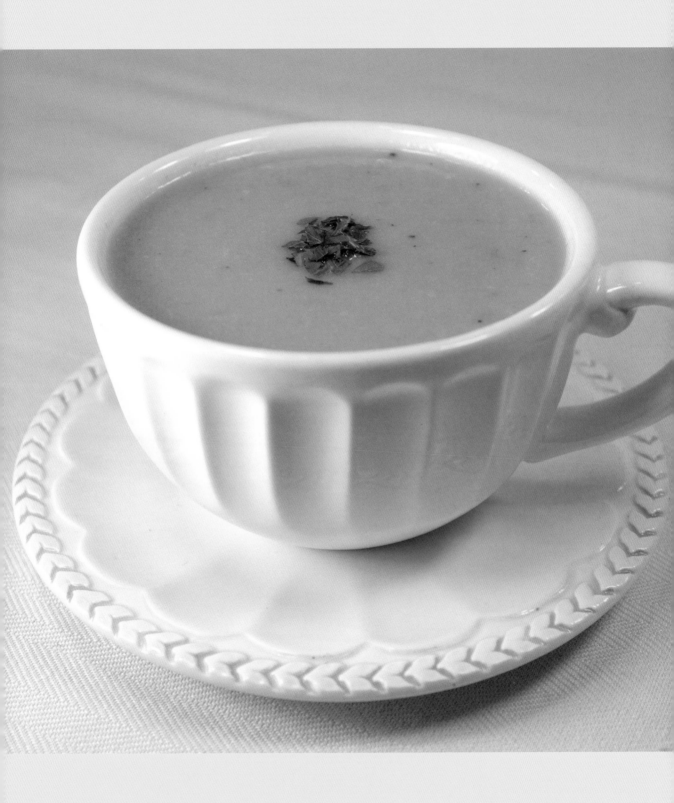

chicken à la king

Using reduced-fat crescent rolls instead of biscuits saves 677 calories per recipe and 30 grams of fat. Definitely worth skipping the biscuits!

½ can (4 rolls) refrigerated reduced-fat crescent roll dough
1 tablespoon butter
1¼ cup cremini mushrooms, sliced
½ green bell pepper, chopped
½ cup low-sodium chicken broth
½ cup frozen peas
2 tablespoons chopped pimento
1½ cups chopped cooked chicken breasts
1 (10¾-ounce) can fat-free condensed cream of mushroom soup
½ cup nonfat milk
Sea salt to taste
Black pepper to taste

1. Prepare the rolls as directed on the package. In a large saucepan over medium heat, melt the butter and add the mushrooms and bell pepper. Sauté until just tender, about 4 minutes. Add the broth, peas, pimento, and chicken. Cook until heated through, about 6 minutes. Whisk in the soup and milk until well combined. Season with salt and pepper as desired.

2. To serve, split the rolls in half and place on serving plates. Spoon the chicken mixture over the rolls and serve.

SERVES 4	
Serving size	1 crescent roll plus ¼ cup sauce

CALORIES PER SERVING	
Original recipe	750
SYS recipe	241

NUTRITIONAL BREAKDOWN	
Fat	11g
Carbohydrates	22g
Protein	16g
Sodium	598mg

trippin' tri-tip tacos

Nonfat cheeses and sour cream are low in calories but still flavorful, and they pair nicely with the fresh herbs and spices of this dish.

1 pound tri-tip

For the marinade:

¼ cup pineapple juice

¼ cup orange juice

1 garlic clove, crushed

¼ teaspoon ground cumin

1 pinch fresh thyme

1 tablespoon Dijon mustard

2 tablespoons low-sodium soy sauce

1 pinch sea salt

1 pinch black pepper

½ teaspoon celery salt

1 tablespoon red chili powder

For the tacos:

1 cup shredded low-fat Cheddar cheese

2 cups shredded iceberg lettuce

2 small tomatoes, diced

½ cup nonfat sour cream

1 small red onion, diced

2 tablespoons chopped fresh cilantro leaves (stems removed)

Hot sauce, as desired

8 taco shells, soft or hard

1. In large mixing bowl, whisk together all the ingredients for the marinade. Immerse the tri-tip in marinade, cover, and refrigerate for 8 hours or overnight. Discard marinade after use. When ready to grill, prepare the taco ingredients by placing them in individual serving bowls.

2. Preheat the grill to medium heat. Grill the marinated tri-tip until the center is medium-rare, or to your desired level of doneness. For medium-rare, allow about 5 minutes of cooking time per 1 inch of thickness. If you do not have an outdoor grill, use a grill pan on the stove top. When ready to serve, thinly slice the steak against the grain.

3. To heat the taco shells, place on a baking sheet in a 225°F oven for about 7 minutes. Assemble the tacos as desired.

SERVES 8		CALORIES PER SERVING		NUTRITIONAL BREAKDOWN	
Serving size	1 taco	Original recipe	424	Fat	12g
		SYS recipe	287	Carbohydrates	25g
				Protein	17g
				Sodium	788mg

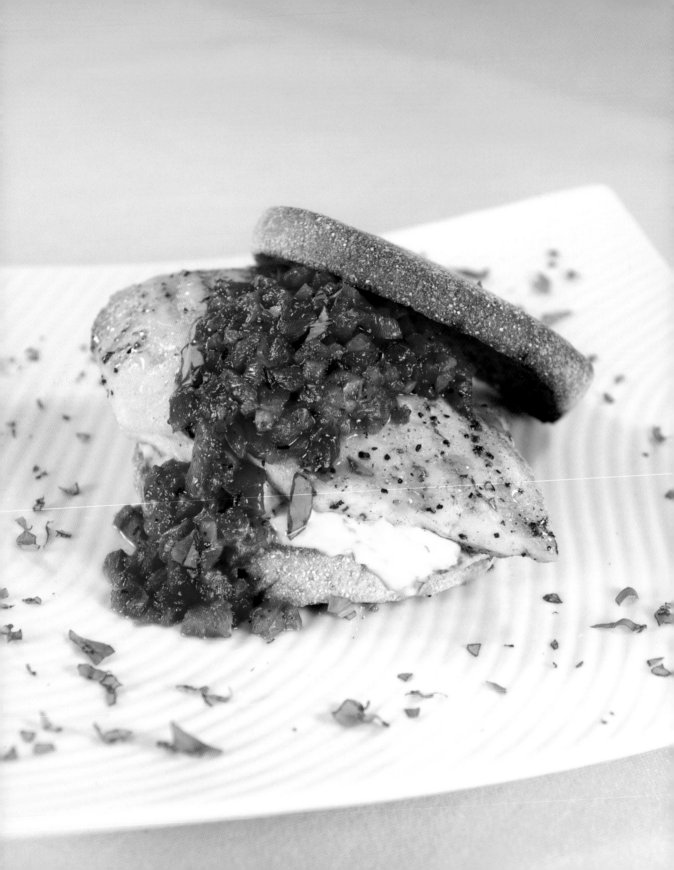

pesto chicken sandwich

High-fiber, high-flavor whole-grain English muffins are a healthy substitution for traditional sourdough rolls or other white flour breads. As well, traditional pesto is loaded with fat and calories due to the heavy oil and nuts. Pack in the basil flavor here and create a new low-calorie, low-fat twist with nonfat mayonnaise and nonfat plain yogurt with a hint of Parmesan cheese.

4 tablespoons nonfat mayonnaise
1 tablespoon nonfat plain yogurt
¼ cup finely chopped fresh basil leaves
1 tablespoon grated Parmesan cheese
4 light multigrain English muffins, lightly toasted
2 (4-ounce) cooked chicken breasts, halved
¼ cup plus 2 tablespoons chopped roasted red bell peppers

1. In a small mixing bowl, mix together the mayonnaise, yogurt, basil, and Parmesan.

2. Assemble the sandwiches by spreading ½ tablespoon mayo mixture on each muffin half (or 1 tablespoon on only the sandwich bottoms, as shown). Top 4 of the muffin halves with chicken breast half, then top each with 1½ tablespoons bell peppers. Finish with the remaining muffin half. Serve.

Skinny Secret

Pesto never tasted so good. For an even lighter sandwich, skip the top muffin half!

SERVES 4	
Serving size	1 sandwich

CALORIES PER SERVING	
Original recipe	479
SYS recipe	234

NUTRITIONAL BREAKDOWN	
Fat	4g
Carbohydrates	27g
Protein	26g
Sodium	405mg

join my club sandwich

Cutting back a little bit in a lot of areas really adds up. Substituting reduced-calorie bread, mayo, and cheese makes a huge difference, as does using lean turkey bacon.

12 slices reduced-calorie wheat bread

6 tablespoons nonfat mayonnaise

½ cup fresh watercress, washed, dried, stems trimmed

8 ounces low-fat deli turkey meat

6 slices lean turkey bacon

4 leaves Boston leaf lettuce, washed, dried, and halved

4 slices tomato, halved

4 slices reduced-fat Swiss cheese, halved

Skinny Secret

Enjoying higher-carb meals earlier in the day gives you needed energy to be productive and allows time for your body to burn it off during the day!

1. Toast the bread and spread ½ tablespoon mayonnaise on each slice of toast. Divide half of the watercress equally among 4 of the bread slices, then add 1 ounce turkey and ¾ slice bacon to each. Top each with a lettuce and tomato half, and then a cheese half. Top each with a slice of bread. Repeat the layering of ingredients, finishing by topping each with a slice of the remaining toast.

2. Secure each sandwich with a toothpick and cut diagonally before serving.

SERVES 4	
Serving size	1 sandwich

CALORIES PER SERVING	
Original recipe	639
SYS recipe	354

NUTRITIONAL BREAKDOWN	
Fat	6g
Carbohydrates	43g
Protein	31g
Sodium	807mg

spice-of-life chili

Ground turkey is much leaner than ground beef—it saves over 15g of fat and 150 calories in this recipe alone!

½ white or yellow onion, chopped

2 cloves garlic, chopped

½ pound lean ground turkey

1 teaspoon chopped fresh oregano

2 tablespoons chili powder

1 (14-ounce) can stewed tomatoes, drained

1 (6-ounce) can tomato paste

5 cups water

1 (15-ounce) can low-sodium kidney beans, drained

In a large-quart boiler over medium heat, combine the onion, garlic, and turkey. Sauté until the turkey is cooked and the onions are tender, about 7 minutes. Stir in the oregano, chili powder, tomatoes, and tomato paste. Stir well, reduce heat to low, and simmer for about 8 minutes. Stir in the water and kidney beans and simmer on low heat for an additional 30 minutes.

Skinny Secret

Chili is flavorful and filling. Most recipes have quite a few ingredients and it takes a little while to make—so go ahead and double the recipe and freeze in individual servings for a quick, healthy meal for lunch or dinner.

SERVES 6		CALORIES PER SERVING		NUTRITIONAL BREAKDOWN	
Serving size	1 cup	Original recipe	460	Fat	5g
		SYS recipe	197	Carbohydrates	22g
				Protein	17g
				Sodium	480mg

chuck wagon chili

Chili is usually served with high-fat cheese. Skip the cheese and use lean beef round steak, fat-free beef broth, and high-protein kidney beans for a muscle-building, low-calorie, low-fat meal.

1 tablespoon olive oil

¾ pound beef round steak, diced into 1-inch cubes

1 white or yellow onion, chopped

3 cloves garlic, chopped

2 cups water

3 cups low-sodium, fat-free beef broth

2 jalapeños, seeded and chopped

2 tablespoons tomato paste

1 tablespoon chili powder

½ tablespoon chopped fresh oregano leaves

1 (15-ounce) can dark red kidney beans, drained and rinsed

1 (15-ounce) can light red kidney beans, drained and rinsed

Sea salt to taste

Black pepper to taste

1. Heat the oil in a large-quart boiler over medium heat. Add the beef, onion, and garlic. Cook until the beef is cooked through, about 7 minutes. Add the water, broth, jalapeño peppers, tomato paste, chili powder, and oregano. Stir well. Add the beans, reduce heat to low, and cover. Simmer for 1 hour, adding broth in ¼ cup increments if needed.

2. When serving, season with salt and pepper as desired.

Skinny Secret

This recipe can be made the day before and kept in the refrigerator. The flavors will actually become more enhanced! Plus, some studies show that eating spicy foods temporarily increases your metabolism, which in turn burns more calories, so spice it up!

SERVES 6		CALORIES PER SERVING		NUTRITIONAL BREAKDOWN	
Serving size	1 cup	Original recipe	477	Fat	10g
		SYS recipe	288	Carbohydrates	32g
				Protein	28g
				Sodium	549mg

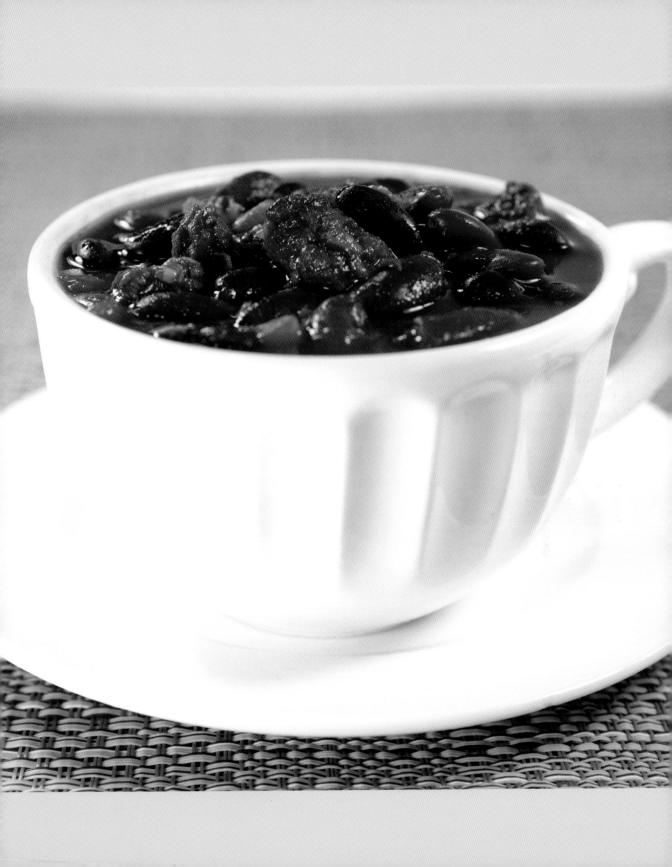

chicken chili

Chicken breasts are naturally lean, and skinless are even leaner! Substituting low-sodium, fat-free chicken broth and reduced-fat Swiss cheese is an easy way to save on calories.

1 tablespoon olive oil

1½ pounds boneless, skinless chicken breasts, finely chopped

2 cloves garlic, chopped

1 small white or yellow onion, chopped

2 cups low-sodium, fat-free chicken broth

2 cups water

1 (15-ounce) can red kidney beans, drained and rinsed

1 (4-ounce) can green chilies

½ cup shredded reduced-fat Swiss cheese

Skinny Secret

Believe it or not, turkey is even leaner than chicken. If you like, substitute ½ pound ground turkey for ½ pound of the chicken and save on 8 grams of fat and 72 calories.

1. In a large-quart boiler, heat the oil over medium heat. Add the chicken, garlic, and onion. Cook until the chicken is cooked through and the onion is tender, about 5 minutes. Add the broth and water, bring to a boil, then reduce heat to low. Stir in the beans and green chilies. Cover and simmer over low heat for about 45 minutes, adding additional chicken broth if needed, in ¼ cup increments.

2. To serve, top with 1 to 1½ tablespoons cheese. Serve hot.

SERVES 4		CALORIES PER SERVING		NUTRITIONAL BREAKDOWN	
Serving size	1 cup	Original recipe	430	Fat	8g
		SYS recipe	259	Carbohydrates	22g
				Protein	24g
				Sodium	510mg

rich french onion soup

CALORIE SAVINGS

144

The fat and calories in French onion soup are in the broth and cheese. Substitute low-sodium, fat-free beef broth and reduced-fat Swiss cheese for the rich flavor you love without the calories.

2 cups thinly sliced white onion

2 tablespoons dry white wine such as sauvignon blanc

4 cups low-sodium, fat-free beef broth

1 teaspoon Worcestershire sauce

4 ounces shredded reduced-fat Swiss cheese

4 slices French bread, toasted

1. In a large-quart boiler over medium heat, combine the onions and wine. Cook until the onions are tender, about 5 to 6 minutes. Add the broth and Worcestershire. Bring to a boil, then reduce heat, cover, and simmer for about 15 minutes.

2. When ready to serve, ladle soup into bowls and top with 1 ounce of the cheese. Float the bread in the bowls or serve on the side, as desired.

Skinny Secret

If you can manage doing without it, skip the bread and save yourself 150 calories and 29g of carbs! Indulge instead in Tropi-Low-Cal Granita for dessert (recipe, page 210).

SERVES 4	
Serving size	1 cup

CALORIES PER SERVING	
Original recipe	375
SYS recipe	231

NUTRITIONAL BREAKDOWN	
Fat	6g
Carbohydrates	34g
Protein	5g
Sodium	387mg

crème de la crème cream of broccoli soup

For any creamed soups, skip the heavy cream and use a potato, which naturally creates a creamy texture.

4 cups water
4 cups broccoli florets
1 baking potato, peeled and cut into 2-inch cubes
1 tablespoon olive oil
1 yellow onion, chopped
1 large stalk celery, chopped
1 cup low-sodium chicken broth
2½ cups nonfat milk
1 pinch ground nutmeg
1 cup nonfat sour cream
Sea salt to taste
Black pepper to taste

1. In a large-quart boiler, combine the water and a pinch of salt. Bring to a boil and add the florets. Allow to boil for 30 seconds. Remove the broccoli and add the potato. Boil until the potato is tender, about 20 minutes. Reserve 1 cup of cooking liquid, then drain.

2. Using the same boiler, heat the olive oil over medium heat. Add the onions and celery, and cook until tender, about 5 minutes. Add the reserved water, broth, and milk. Whisk in the nutmeg and sour cream until smooth. Add the potatoes and ¾ of the broccoli. Reduce heat and simmer until heated through, stirring occasionally. Do not boil. Season with salt and pepper.

3. Working in batches, purée in a food processor until smooth. To serve, ladle 1-cup portions into bowls and distribute the remaining florets equally among the serving bowls.

SERVES 6	
Serving size	1 cup

CALORIES PER SERVING	
Original recipe	342
SYS recipe	140

NUTRITIONAL BREAKDOWN	
Fat	3g
Carbohydrates	22g
Protein	8g
Sodium	139mg

creamy tomato soup

Creamed soups get their creaminess from high-calorie and high-fat heavy whipping cream or half-and-half. Using low-sodium juice, nonfat milk, and nonfat sour cream are perfect substitutions for this low-calorie creamed soup.

4 large tomatoes, seeded and diced
4 cups low-sodium V-8 juice or similar low-sodium tomato juice
1 large shallot, chopped
½ cup coarsely chopped fresh basil leaves
½ cup nonfat milk
½ cup nonfat sour cream
Sea salt to taste
Black pepper to taste

1. In a large-quart boiler over medium-high heat, combine the tomatoes, tomato juice, and shallot. Heat to just before the boiling point. Reduce heat to a simmer, cover, and let simmer for about 25 minutes. Stir in the basil, milk, and sour cream; simmer for an additional 5 minutes, or until heated through. Season with salt and pepper.

2. Working in batches, purée the mixture in a food processor or blender until smooth. Ladle 1-cup servings into bowls. Serve hot or chilled.

Skinny Secret

High-sodium foods make you retain water, leaving you feeling bloated and uncomfortable. When possible, use low-sodium products and drink lots of water to relieve that bloated feeling.

SERVES 4	
Serving size	1 cup

CALORIES PER SERVING	
Original recipe	475
SYS recipe	105

NUTRITIONAL BREAKDOWN	
Fat	1g
Carbohydrates	21g
Protein	5g
Sodium	203mg

potato and leek soup

As with most creamy soups, skip the cream. Since this recipe is used with potatoes, you need no cream at all.

4 baking potatoes, peeled and cut into 1-inch cubes
5 cups low-sodium, fat-free chicken broth
1 tablespoon butter
2 leeks, bulb only, cleaned and sliced
¼ cup dry white wine such as sauvignon blanc
Sea salt to taste
White pepper to taste

Skinny Secret

Other delicious vegetables that work well instead of leeks in this recipe include broccoli, asparagus, or roasted red peppers. They're all equally lean.

1. In a large-quart boiler, combine the potatoes and chicken broth. If needed, add water so that the potatoes are covered with liquid. Bring to a boil and boil until tender, about 20 minutes. Drain, reserving 2 cups of the liquid. Working in batches, purée the potatoes with ¼ cup of the liquid. Return the puréed potatoes to the boiler.

2. In a medium saucepan, melt the butter over medium heat. Add the leeks and sauté for about 2 minutes. Add the wine, and season with salt and pepper. Sauté for an additional 2 minutes. Stir the leeks into the potato mixture. Mix well. Bring to a simmer, adding the reserved water as needed to thin out the soup to the desired consistency. Cook until heated through, but do not boil the soup. Season with salt and pepper to taste. Serve in 1-cup portions.

SERVES 10	
Serving size	¾ cup

CALORIES PER SERVING	
Original recipe	423
SYS recipe	83

NUTRITIONAL BREAKDOWN	
Fat	1g
Carbohydrates	15g
Protein	2g
Sodium	35mg

not-so-fat tuesday gumbo

Increasing flavorful, healthy vegetables, substituting turkey sausage for traditional high-fat sausage, and using it in combination with a lower amount of higher-fat andouille sausage keeps the fat out of this recipe. For added fiber, substitute whole-grain brown rice for the white rice.

1 tablespoon olive oil

1 white or yellow onion, chopped

1 jalapeño, seeded and minced

1 red bell pepper, diced

1 green bell pepper, diced

3 cloves garlic, diced

1 andouille sausage, chopped

¼ pound turkey sausage, chopped

1 (1-pound) package frozen mixed vegetables

1 (32-ounce) can diced tomatoes

1 teaspoon paprika

1 teaspoon chili powder

1 teaspoon cayenne pepper

2 teaspoons Worcestershire sauce

2 cups low-sodium chicken broth

1 cup water

2 cups cooked white rice

In a large-quart boiler, heat the olive oil over medium heat. Add the onion, jalapeño, bell peppers, and garlic. Sauté until tender, about 5 minutes. Add the andouille and turkey sausage and cook until browned, about 6 minutes. Add the vegetables, tomatoes, paprika, chili powder, cayenne, and Worcestershire. Reduce heat and simmer for about 7 minutes. Add the broth and water, cover, and simmer for about 25 minutes, stirring occasionally. Stir in the rice and cook for an additional 10 minutes. When ready to serve, ladle 1 cup into each serving bowl. Enjoy.

Skinny Secret

Gumbo is a very filling style of soup and is great for lunch or dinner. Make this recipe for yourself and store in individual servings in the freezer for a quick, easy, low-calorie meal.

SERVES 6	
Serving size	1 cup

CALORIES PER SERVING	
Original recipe	460
SYS recipe	189

NUTRITIONAL BREAKDOWN	
Fat	5g
Carbohydrates	27g
Protein	8g
Sodium	455mg

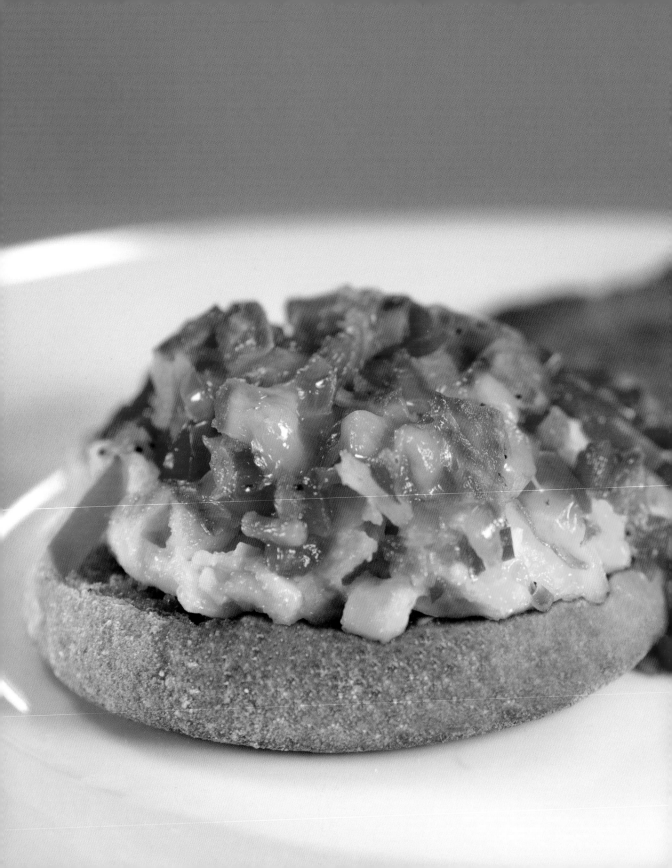

western-style sandwich

Turkey ham, whole-grain English muffins, and reduced-fat jack cheese cut down on calories, add much needed dietary fiber, and still taste great. Cooking with nonfat spray instead of butter is another simple way to keep recipes lean.

1 tablespoon olive oil
½ white or yellow onion, chopped
½ red bell pepper, diced
½ green bell pepper, diced
2 slices turkey ham, chopped
Nonstick cooking spray
2 eggs, beaten
Sea salt
Black pepper
2 light whole-grain English muffins
2 tablespoons reduced-fat Monterey jack cheese

1. In skillet or saucepan, heat the olive oil on medium. Add the onion and red and green bell peppers. Sauté until tender, about 5 minutes. Add the turkey ham and cook until heated through. Transfer to a bowl and cover with plastic wrap.

2. Using the same skillet, spray lightly, if needed, with nonstick spray. Heat on medium. Add the eggs and scramble until just cooked.

3. Place the English muffin halves on serving plates. Top each with half of the egg mixture and half of the onion mixture. Season with salt and pepper as desired. Top each with 1 tablespoon cheese, and finish with the remaining muffin half. Serve.

Skinny Secret

Add additional flavor without adding too many calories and virtually no fat by adding a tablespoon or two of freshly chopped broccoli florets, asparagus tips, or fresh tomatoes. If you do add them, sauté them with the onions and peppers.

SERVES 2		CALORIES PER SERVING		NUTRITIONAL BREAKDOWN	
Serving size	1 sandwich	Original recipe	530	Fat	15g
		SYS recipe	286	Carbohydrates	31g
				Protein	30g
				Sodium	638mg

roasty toasty beef sandwich

Substitute nonfat mayonnaise and reduced-fat Monterey jack cheese for instant calorie savings. However, commit to portion control by enjoying only one slice of bread per serving instead of the traditional two.

3 tablespoons nonfat mayonnaise

2 teaspoons prepared horseradish

1 tablespoon olive oil

1 yellow onion, thinly sliced

2 ciabatta rolls, halved

4 ounces deli roast beef

4 thin slices reduced-fat Monterey jack cheese

Skinny Secret

If you prefer a "bottom" and a "top" to your sandwich, substitute a low-fat, reduced-calorie English muffin for the ciabatta bread.

1. In a small mixing bowl, combine the mayonnaise and horseradish. Mix well and set aside.

2. In a medium sauté pan, heat the oil over medium-low heat. Add the onions and sauté until very tender and turning slightly browned, about 15 minutes. Add 2 tablespoons of water, if needed, to prevent burning, and sauté for an additional 3 minutes.

3. Preheat the broiler. Spread ¾ tablespoon of the horseradish mixture on each ciabatta half. Equally divide the sautéed onions among the 4 halves. Top each with 1 slice of roast beef and 1 slice of cheese. Place under the broiler until the cheese melts. Serve hot.

4. This recipe serves ½ of each ciabatta roll as a serving, using both top half and bottom half of roll as the base for the sandwich.

SERVES 4		CALORIES PER SERVING		NUTRITIONAL BREAKDOWN	
Serving size	1 sandwich	Original recipe	675	Fat	7g
		SYS recipe	271	Carbohydrates	29g
				Protein	21g
				Sodium	554mg

thinner dinners

summer savoring
mac 'n' cheese

Mac 'n' cheese is a family favorite! Keep it lean by using nonfat ricotta and reduced-fat sharp Cheddar cheeses!

Nonstick cooking spray
8 ounces dried macaroni
¾ cup nonfat ricotta cheese
½ cup reduced-fat sharp Cheddar cheese
1 tablespoon chopped fresh basil leaves
1 (14-ounce) can diced tomatoes, drained
Sea salt and pepper to taste

Skinny Secret

Mac 'n' cheese tastes so good, you might eat spoonfuls before even getting it to the dinner plate, thereby causing you to overeat. To avoid that, keep smaller individual-serving-size dishes next to the stove so you can transfer it directly from oven to table.

Preheat oven to 350°F. Spray a small baking dish with nonstick spray. Prepare the macaroni according to package directions. In a medium saucepan over medium-low heat, combine the ricotta and Cheddar cheese. Stir until the cheese is melted and well mixed. Add the basil and tomatoes, then season with salt and pepper. Mix with the prepared macaroni. Transfer to small baking dish, cover with aluminum foil, and bake for 15 to 20 minutes.

SERVES 4	
Serving size	½ cup

CALORIES PER SERVING	
Original recipe	320
SYS recipe	254

NUTRITIONAL BREAKDOWN	
Fat	8g
Carbohydrates	50g
Protein	14g
Sodium	187mg

skinny "beef" stroganoff

Substituting lean ground turkey for beef is one of the best ways to decrease fat and calories (plus it tastes great!). The other substitution here is nonfat sour cream, which gives a creamy texture to the dish, not your waistline!

8 ounces dried egg noodles
½ cup ground turkey
½ white onion, chopped
½ cup chopped cremini mushrooms
¼ cup chopped celery
¾ cup nonfat sour cream
Sea salt and black pepper to taste

1. Prepare the egg noodles as directed on the package. Drain and reserve ¾ cup of the liquid.

2. In a large saucepan over medium heat, cook the turkey and onion until the turkey is browned and the onion is tender, about 5 minutes. Drain and return to the saucepan. Add ½ cup of the liquid from the noodles, the mushrooms, and celery. Cook until the celery is tender, about 5 minutes. Add the sour cream and stir until well combined. Add the remaining ¼ cup of liquid from the noodles if needed. Season with salt and pepper. Stir in the noodles and serve.

Skinny Secret

Lean, chopped, cooked chicken breasts are a delicious alternative to beef and ground turkey.

SERVES 4	
Serving size	½ cup

CALORIES PER SERVING	
Original recipe	390
SYS recipe	294

NUTRITIONAL BREAKDOWN	
Fat	6g
Carbohydrates	45g
Protein	14g
Sodium	84mg

lean, mean meatloaf

Nonstick cooking spray allows you to cook without adding calories of oil and butter. You can buy butter-flavored nonstick spray if you want extra butter flavor; however, I don't recommend it for this recipe.

Nonstick cooking spray
1 tablespoon olive oil
⅓ cup chopped cremini mushrooms
¼ cup chopped white onion
1 clove garlic, minced
1 egg
1 tablespoon nonfat milk
½ teaspoon sea salt
½ teaspoon ground black pepper
½ tablespoon chopped fresh basil leaves
½ tablespoon chopped fresh Italian flat-leaf parsley
¼ cup dry bread crumbs, plain or seasoned
½ pound lean ground turkey
¼ cup ketchup (optional)

Skinny Secret

A good way to measure portion size is to use the size of your fist as a guide. The size of your fist is equal to about 4 to 5 ounces of food, which is the optimum serving size for nearly all foods.

1. Preheat oven to 350°F. Prepare a small loaf pan by spraying with nonstick cooking spray. In a heavy skillet, heat the olive oil over medium heat. Add the mushrooms, onion, and garlic. Sauté until the garlic is fragrant and the onion is tender, about 3 to 4 minutes. Remove from heat and set aside.

2. In a small bowl, whisk together the egg and milk. Add the salt, pepper, basil, and parsley. Whisk together. Add the bread crumbs and stir to combine. Add the turkey and the mushroom mixture, and mix well. Gently press the mixture into a loaf pan, cover with aluminum foil, and bake for 35 minutes.

3. Uncover and cook for an additional 5 to 10 minutes or until a thermometer reads 165°F. Optional: Just before baking uncovered, spread ¼ cup ketchup on top of the meatloaf and then finish baking.

SERVES 4		CALORIES PER SERVING		NUTRITIONAL BREAKDOWN	
Serving size	½ cup	Original recipe	240	Fat	12g
		SYS recipe	142	Carbohydrates	5g
				Protein	8g
				Sodium	80mg

chicken alfredo

Nonfat milk and nonfat sour cream are the perfect substitution for fat-laden heavy cream and give you the high-flavor creaminess you look for in Alfredo sauces. Lean skinless chicken breasts are excellent for adding protein.

8 ounces dried fettuccini pasta
1 tablespoon butter
½ white or yellow onion, chopped
1 clove garlic, chopped
2 tablespoons plain flour
½ cup nonfat milk
½ cup nonfat sour cream
¼ cup grated Parmesan cheese
1 teaspoon crushed red pepper flakes
1 cup chopped cooked chicken breasts
1 tablespoon chopped fresh Italian flat-leaf parsley
Sea salt to taste
Black pepper to taste

Skinny Secret

You can also substitute lean turkey breast, which is lower in both calories and fat.

1. Prepare the fettuccini as directed on the package. In a large saucepan, melt the butter over medium heat. Add the onion and garlic and sauté until just tender, about 4 minutes. Add the flour and stir to form a slight paste. Whisk in the milk and sour cream. Bring to a boil, reduce heat, and let simmer for 2 minutes, stirring often. Whisk in the Parmesan cheese and red pepper flakes, and stir to combine. Add the chicken and parsley, and stir well. Season with salt and pepper.

2. To serve, place 1 cup fettuccini on each serving plate and top with ¼ cup sauce.

SERVES 4	
Serving size	1 cup pasta and ¼ cup sauce

CALORIES PER SERVING	
Original recipe	990
SYS recipe	351

NUTRITIONAL BREAKDOWN	
Fat	7g
Carbohydrates	50g
Protein	23g
Sodium	167mg

fettuccini alfredo

Most of the fat in fettuccini Alfredo is in the heavy cream and cheese. Substituting nonfat milk and nonfat sour cream for the heavy cream saves a load of fat and calories, as does reduced-fat ricotta. Each of these ingredients, however, still provides you the creaminess you love in traditional Alfredo dishes.

8 ounces dried fettuccini pasta
1 tablespoon butter
2 garlic cloves, finely chopped
2 teaspoons plain flour
1⅓ cup nonfat milk
2 tablespoons nonfat sour cream
¼ cup reduced-fat ricotta cheese
½ cup grated Parmesan cheese
1 pinch nutmeg
½ teaspoon black pepper

Skinny Secret

Try to eat pasta earlier in the day so your body will have time to burn off the calories and carbs.

1. Prepare the pasta as directed on the package. In a medium saucepan, heat the butter on medium and add the garlic. Sauté until fragrant, about 1 minute. Whisk in the flour and cook until a slight paste is formed. Whisk in the milk, sour cream, ricotta cheese, and Parmesan cheese. Combine well and bring to a boil, then reduce heat. Simmer for 2 minutes while whisking continually until it thickens slightly. Add the nutmeg and pepper. Remove from heat.

2. To serve, place 1 cup pasta on each plate and top with ¼ cup sauce. Garnish with chopped Italian flat-leaf parsley, if desired.

SERVES 4	
Serving size	1 cup pasta and ¼ cup sauce

CALORIES PER SERVING	
Original recipe	500
SYS recipe	351

NUTRITIONAL BREAKDOWN	
Fat	8g
Carbohydrates	52g
Protein	17g
Sodium	299mg

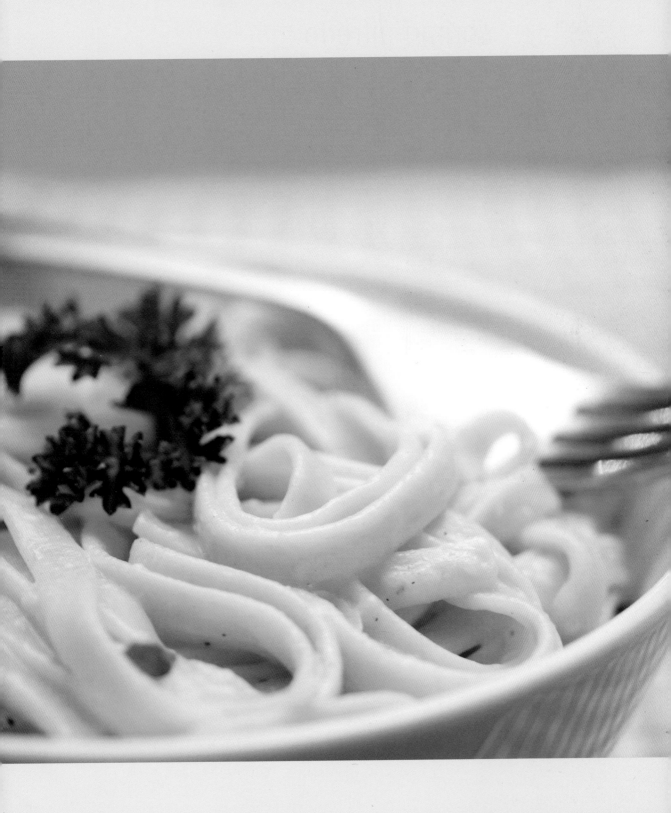

shrimp alfredo

As suggested in both the traditional Fettuccini Alfredo and the Chicken Alfredo recipes, a combination of nonfat milk and nonfat sour cream are great for reducing fat and calories normally found in heavy cream sauces. This shrimp version is a delicious alternative to chicken and gets maximum flavor from the added herbs and spices.

8 ounces dried fettuccini pasta

2 tablespoons butter

1 clove garlic, minced

½ white or yellow onion, chopped

2 tablespoons plain flour

2 cups nonfat milk

½ cup nonfat sour cream

1 teaspoon hot pepper sauce

¼ cup grated Parmesan cheese

1 cup cooked bay shrimp

1 tablespoon chopped fresh Italian flat-leaf parsley

Sea salt to taste

Black pepper to taste

Skinny Secret

You can also use scallops, clams, mussels, or cooked lobster in this recipe.

1. Prepare the pasta as directed on the package. In a large saucepan over medium heat, melt the butter. Add the garlic and onion and sauté for about 4 minutes, until tender. Stir in the flour to form a light paste. Whisk in the milk and sour cream. Bring to a boil, reduce heat, and let simmer for about 2 minutes, stirring often. Stir in the hot sauce and Parmesan cheese. Stir well to combine. Add the shrimp and parsley. Season with salt and pepper. Stir well and cook until heated through, about 2 minutes.

2. Serve 1 cup pasta with ¼ cup sauce on each dinner plate.

SERVES 4		CALORIES PER SERVING		NUTRITIONAL BREAKDOWN	
Serving size	1 cup pasta with ¼ cup sauce	Original recipe	776	Fat	9g
		SYS recipe	410	Carbohydrates	55g
				Protein	27g
				Sodium	327mg

sweet-and-sour chicken

CALORIE SAVINGS

82

Sweet-and-sour chicken can be loaded with sugary calories. Keep this dish lean and flavorful by using skinless chicken breasts, egg white, reducing the amount of sugar and oil used, and using the natural juices of the pineapple and mandarin oranges to create that sweet flavor you love while keeping calories down.

1 pound boneless, skinless chicken breasts, cut into 1-inch pieces

1 egg white

½ teaspoon sea salt

2 teaspoons cornstarch

1 (10-ounce) can pineapple chunks, juice reserved

1 (10-ounce) can mandarin oranges, juice reserved

¼ cup apple cider vinegar

¼ cup ketchup

2 tablespoons brown sugar

2 tablespoons canola oil

1 red bell pepper, cut into 1-inch chunks

1 yellow bell pepper, cut into 1-inch chunks

1 teaspoon grated fresh gingerroot

1. In a medium mixing bowl, combine the chicken with the egg white, salt, and cornstarch. Toss to coat the chicken evenly. Let rest for 15 minutes.

2. Whisk together 2 tablespoons of the pineapple juice and 2 table-spoons of the mandarin orange juice. Discard the remaining juice. Whisk the vinegar, ketchup, and brown sugar with the juice mixture.

3. Heat a large sauté pan over medium-high heat and add 1 tablespoon of the oil. When the oil is hot, add the chicken, spreading it out in the pan to cook evenly. Let the chicken fry for 1 minute, until browned. Stir and cook for an additional minute until browned on all sides. Remove the chicken from the pan and set aside.

4. Reduce heat to medium and add the remaining tablespoon of oil. Add the bell peppers and gingerroot. Cook for 2 minutes, stirring occasionally. Add the pineapple chunks and oranges along with the juice mixture. Turn heat to high and let simmer for about 1 minute. Add the chicken and continue to simmer for about 2 minutes. Serve as is or over cooked rice.

SERVES 4		CALORIES PER SERVING		NUTRITIONAL BREAKDOWN	
Serving size	1 cup	Original recipe	450	Fat	12g
		SYS recipe	368	Carbohydrates	30g
				Protein	38g
				Sodium	248mg

buff 'n' low buffalo chicken chowder

Buffalo wings are usually cooked with the skin on, which is where most of the fat is. Combining wing sauce with nonfat cream of celery soup and fresh cilantro is a great way to enjoy the flavor of buffalo wings while saving on the fat. Traditional wings have an average of 100 calories per wing and up to 23 grams of fat; yikes!

1 tablespoon butter
1 white or yellow onion, chopped
6 cups nonfat milk
1 cup nonfat sour cream
3 (10¾-ounce) cans fat-free condensed cream of celery soup
3 cups shredded cooked chicken breasts
¼ cup chopped fresh cilantro leaves
½ cup buffalo wing sauce (such as Red Hot)
Sea salt to taste

1. In a large-quart boiler, melt the butter over medium heat and add the onion. Sauté until tender, about 4 minutes. Add the milk, sour cream, soup, chicken, cilantro, and wing sauce. Stir to combine. Bring to a boil, then reduce heat to low, and simmer for 45 minutes, adding water if needed to prevent drying.

2. When ready, season with salt to taste. Serve in bowls in 1-cup portions.

SERVES 8		CALORIES PER SERVING		NUTRITIONAL BREAKDOWN	
Serving size	1 cup	Original recipe	490	Fat	6g
		SYS recipe	239	Carbohydrates	21g
				Protein	24g
				Sodium	609mg

teriyummy beef

CALORIE
SAVINGS
250

Lean cuts of beef, fresh natural juice, and cutting back on sugar and oil all combine to make this a truly light and flavorful dish that is perfect for lunch or dinner.

1 cup low-sodium soy sauce

2 tablespoons canola oil

2 tablespoons rice wine vinegar

2 tablespoons brown sugar

½ teaspoon ground ginger

½ teaspoon garlic powder

Fine zest of ¼ orange

1 tablespoon fresh orange juice

1 tablespoon sherry wine

¾ pound beef round steak, cut into 1-inch cubes

1 tablespoon water

1. In a medium mixing bowl, whisk together the soy sauce, oil, vinegar, sugar, ginger, garlic powder, orange zest, orange juice, and sherry. Whisk well to combine. Transfer to a sealable plastic bag and add the beef cubes. Seal the bag tightly and shake to coat. Refrigerate for at least 1 hour, or overnight.

2. When ready to cook, remove the beef from the bag and discard any remaining marinade. Heat a sauté pan over medium heat. Add the beef and 1 tablespoon water. Cover, reduce heat to low, and simmer for 5 to 7 minutes, or until the beef is cooked through. Serve as is or over cooked rice.

Skinny Secret

This marinade is also great with chicken and lean pork! Drink lots of water when enjoying this recipe, as the sodium content is high even in low-sodium soy sauce.

SERVES 4	
Serving size	1 cup

CALORIES PER SERVING	
Original recipe	520
SYS recipe	270

NUTRITIONAL BREAKDOWN	
Fat	13g
Carbohydrates	10g
Protein	29g
Sodium	2,180mg

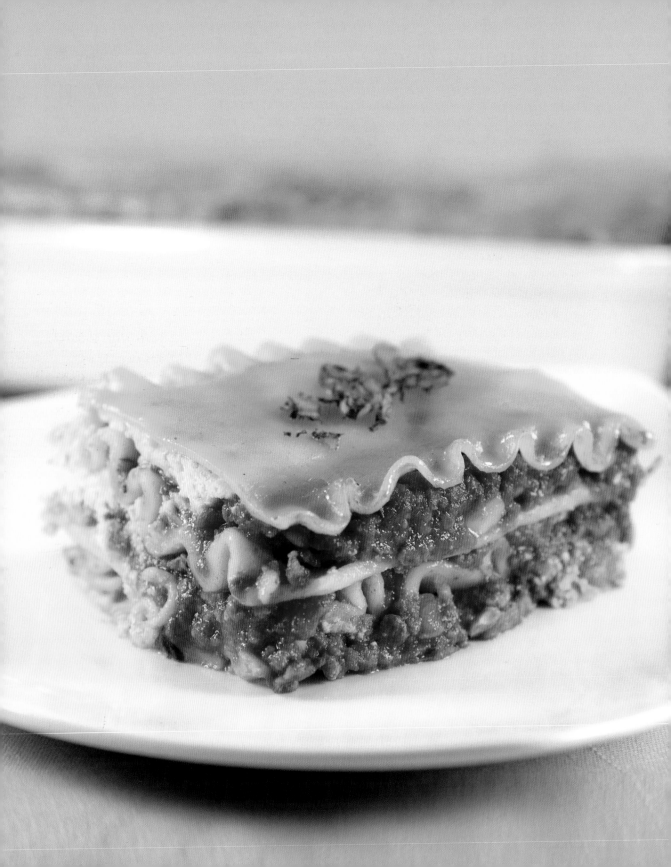

i'm feelin' lazy lasagna

When cooking any kind of ground beef recipe, go for the leanest ground beef—98 percent fat-free. This gives you a lean base to begin with; substituting nonfat ricotta and cottage cheeses keeps your lasagna even lighter.

1 pound dried lasagna noodles

1 tablespoon olive oil

1 white or yellow onion, chopped

2 cloves garlic, chopped

¾ pound lean ground beef

2 teaspoons chopped fresh oregano leaves

1 tablespoon chopped fresh basil leaves

2 teaspoons chopped fresh Italian flat-leaf parsley leaves

½ cup chopped cremini mushrooms

1 (28-ounce) can diced tomatoes

2 (6-ounce) cans tomato paste

1 cup water

Sea salt to taste

Black pepper to taste

2 cups nonfat ricotta cheese

1 cup nonfat cottage cheese

¼ cup grated Parmesan cheese

Nonstick cooking spray

Skinny Secret

For an even lighter lasagna, substitute lean ground turkey for the beef and skip the top layer of lasagna noodles.

1. Preheat oven to 400°F. Prepare the lasagna noodles as directed on the package. When cooked and drained, drizzle with olive oil to prevent sticking.

continued

SERVES 12		CALORIES PER SERVING		NUTRITIONAL BREAKDOWN	
Serving size	½₂ of lasagna, about 1 cup	Original recipe	580	Fat	3g
		SYS recipe	272	Carbohydrates	42g
				Protein	19g
				Sodium	365mg

i'm feelin' lazy lasagna

continued

2. In a large saucepan over medium heat, add the onion, garlic, and beef. Sauté until the beef is browned and the onion is tender, about 7 minutes. Drain off the grease. Add the oregano, basil, parsley, mushrooms, tomatoes, tomato paste, and water. Stir to mix well. Season with salt and pepper. Reduce heat to low and simmer for about 25 minutes.

3. In a medium mixing bowl, combine the ricotta, cottage cheese, and Parmesan. Mix well.

4. To make the lasagna, prepare a deep, rectangular baking dish by spraying it with nonstick spray. Arrange the lasagna noodles in a single layer on the bottom of the pan. Spread with ⅓ of the meat sauce. Top with ⅓ of the cheese mixture. Add another layer of lasagna noodles and top with half of the remaining meat mixture and half of the remaining cheese mixture. Repeat with another layer of noodles, using the remaining meat and cheese mixtures. Finish with a layer of noodles on top.

5. Cover with foil and bake for 1 hour and 20 minutes. Remove from the oven and let rest for about 15 minutes. Cut into 12 portions and serve.

6. *Note:* For ease in serving, arrange bottom layer of noodles horizontally, trimming as needed. Then, when adding the next layer of noodles, arrange vertically. Continue alternating the direction of the noodles as you complete the recipe. This will help hold the lasagna together when serving.

parmesan chicken

Parmesan chicken has fat and calories oozing at the seams. Substitute skinless chicken breasts, egg whites for whole eggs, nonfat cheeses for full-fat versions, and cook with nonfat cooking spray to reduce unwanted calories and keep you slim and trim.

3 egg whites, lightly beaten

2 cups Italian-style bread crumbs

4 boneless, skinless chicken breasts, about 4 ounces each

¼ cup nonfat mozzarella cheese

¼ cup nonfat ricotta cheese

1⅓ cups meatless spaghetti sauce

Nonstick cooking spray

1. Preheat oven to 375°F. Spray a 9" × 13" baking dish with nonstick spray. Place the egg whites in a medium bowl and the bread crumbs in a separate medium bowl. Dip the chicken in the egg whites, then coat with bread crumbs. In a medium bowl, combine the mozzarella and ricotta cheese. Mix well.

2. Spray a medium skillet with nonstick spray and heat on medium. Add the coated chicken to the pan and brown on each side, about 4 minutes per side. Transfer the chicken to the prepared baking dish and top each with ⅓ cup of spaghetti sauce. Top with ¼ cup of the cheese mixture. Cover the dish with foil and bake for 20 minutes. Uncover and bake for an additional 5 minutes or until done.

Skinny Secret

To serve this as an appetizer, slice the chicken into 1-inch-thick strips and prepare as directed. The baking time will be less, about 7 minutes total in the oven.

SERVES 4		CALORIES PER SERVING		NUTRITIONAL BREAKDOWN	
Serving size	1 cup	Original recipe	717	Fat	4g
		SYS recipe	256	Carbohydrates	10g
				Protein	28g
				Sodium	805mg

meatball mania spaghetti

Baking the meatballs as opposed to pan-frying saves over 360 calories and 42 grams of fat!

½ pound lean ground turkey
¼ cup quick-cooking oats
1 egg white
½ teaspoon dried oregano
¼ teaspoon dried thyme
½ teaspoon dried basil
½ teaspoon sea salt
½ teaspoon black pepper
1 cup low-sodium spaghetti sauce
8 ounces dried spaghetti noodles

1. Preheat oven to 400°F. In a large mixing bowl, combine the turkey, oats, egg, oregano, thyme, basil, salt, and pepper. Mix well. Roll into 12 meatballs (about 1 heaping tablespoon each). Spray a heavy ovenproof skillet with nonstick spray. Place the meatballs in skillet and bake for 12 minutes or until done.

2. In a medium skillet, warm the sauce over medium heat until heated through, about 5 minutes.

3. Prepare the spaghetti as directed on the package. When ready to serve, place 1 cup of pasta on each plate, and top each with ¼ cup sauce and 3 meatballs.

SERVES 4	
Serving size	3 meatballs with ¼ cup sauce and 1 cup pasta

CALORIES PER SERVING	
Original recipe	542
SYS recipe	402

NUTRITIONAL BREAKDOWN	
Fat	9g
Carbohydrates	48g
Protein	30g
Sodium	367mg

hottie-tottie manicotti

Keep your figure slim by substituting reduced-fat and nonfat cheeses as well as low-fat pasta sauce. Not only are the cheeses still flavorful, but the fresh basil and oregano add delicious flavor without adding fat or calories. Spraying your baking dish with nonstick spray is a great way to prevent sticking and at the same time eliminate extra calories and fat.

8 ounces dried manicotti shells
1 tablespoon olive oil
1 cup shredded reduced-fat mozzarella cheese
1 cup reduced-fat ricotta cheese
1 cup nonfat cottage cheese
¼ cup grated Parmesan cheese
½ cup chopped fresh basil leaves
1 teaspoon chopped fresh oregano leaves
½ teaspoon sea salt
1 teaspoon black pepper
1 (26-ounce) jar meatless low-fat pasta sauce
Nonstick cooking spray

1. Prepare the manicotti as directed on the package. Preheat oven to 400°F. Spray a rectangular baking dish with nonstick spray. When the manicotti is ready, drain and drizzle with the olive oil. Gently toss to coat.

2. Prepare the filling by combining the mozzarella, ricotta, cottage cheese, and Parmesan. Mix well and add the basil, oregano, salt, and pepper. Mix to blend. Stuff 2 tablespoons of mixture into each shell.

3. Spread ½ cup sauce in the bottom of the prepared baking dish. Layer with the filled shells. Top with any remaining cheese and the sauce. Cover the dish with foil and bake for 30 minutes. Uncover and bake for an additional 10 to 15 minutes. Serve hot.

Skinny Secret

This is a dish that freezes well. Just be sure to freeze in individual portions to avoid thawing and refreezing the entire dish. If desired, add 2 cups cooked lean ground turkey to the pasta sauce, which adds an additional 53 calories per serving.

SERVES 10	
Serving size	1 cup

CALORIES PER SERVING	
Original recipe	942
SYS recipe	250

NUTRITIONAL BREAKDOWN	
Fat	7g
Carbohydrates	30g
Protein	16g
Sodium	656mg

peppery chicken pasta

Lemon chicken is usually served with a heavy cream sauce. Cooking the chicken in the lemon adds flavor without adding fat and calories. Substituting olive oil for the heavy cream keeps this recipe light and tasty.

4 ounces dried penne pasta
½ tablespoon plus 3 tablespoons olive oil
3 (4-ounce) boneless, skinless chicken breasts
½ cup water
1 lemon, juiced and sliced
1 teaspoon red pepper flakes
¼ cup grated Parmesan cheese
Sea salt to taste
Black pepper to taste

Skinny Secret

You can substitute turkey for chicken in this dish if you prefer.

1. Prepare the penne pasta as directed on the package. Drain and toss with ½ tablespoon of the olive oil. In a medium sauté pan, cook the chicken, water, lemon juice, and lemon slices over medium heat. Cover and reduce heat to medium-low. Simmer for about 10 minutes or until the chicken is cooked through, turning once.

2. Toss the pasta with the remaining olive oil, the red pepper flakes, and cheese. Season with salt and pepper. Slice the chicken breasts. Divide the pasta mixture into 4 equal portions. Top each serving with chicken and lemon slices.

SERVES 4	
Serving size	1 cup

CALORIES PER SERVING	
Original recipe	528
SYS recipe	327

NUTRITIONAL BREAKDOWN	
Fat	20g
Carbohydrates	22g
Protein	22g
Sodium	112mg

monterey chicken

CALORIE SAVINGS

345

Turkey bacon, skinless chicken breasts, sugar-free BBQ sauce, and reduced-fat cheese are all great ways to cut back on calories. It all adds up to substantial savings per serving!

2 slices turkey bacon

4 (4-ounce) boneless, skinless chicken breasts

Sea salt to taste

Black pepper to taste

½ cup water

¼ cup sugar-free barbecue sauce

½ cup shredded reduced-fat Monterey jack cheese

4 red lettuce leaves, washed and dried

1. Preheat broiler. In a large ovenproof skillet over medium heat, cook the bacon until crisp. Drain on paper towels. Lightly season the chicken with salt and pepper. Return skillet to heat and add the chicken and water. Cover and reduce heat to medium-low. Cook until the chicken is cooked through, about 15 to 18 minutes, turning once.

2. Remove the chicken from the skillet; toss with the barbecue sauce. Return to the skillet, top with the cheese, and place under the broiler. Broil until the cheese is just melted. Place a lettuce leaf on each serving plate and top each with a chicken breast and half a bacon slice.

Skinny Secret

Make a true salad out of this recipe by cutting the cooked chicken into 1-inch cubes, crumbling the bacon, and tossing them with the cheese and greens. For dressing, drizzle with 1 tablespoon of fresh lemon juice, or if you must have real dressing, use fat-free Italian.

SERVES 4	
Serving size	1 cup

CALORIES PER SERVING	
Original recipe	642
SYS recipe	297

NUTRITIONAL BREAKDOWN	
Fat	18g
Carbohydrates	3.5g
Protein	43g
Sodium	507mg

smokin-good bacon burger

Lean proteins such as turkey bacon and lean ground beef are perfect for reducing fat and calories. Substitute one egg white for a whole egg and place it all on a high-fiber whole-grain bun for a burger that's high in flavor and nutrients and low in calories.

2 slices turkey bacon
¾ pound lean ground beef
1 teaspoon Worcestershire sauce
1 egg, lightly beaten
1 egg white, lightly beaten
Sea salt (about 1 teaspoon)
Black pepper (about 1 teaspoon)
1 teaspoon garlic powder
¼ cup white or yellow onion, minced
4 whole-grain hamburger buns

Skinny Secret

This burger is flavorful on its own, so skip the mayo and ketchup and use toppings such as a fresh slice of tomato, lettuce leaf, and even a few fresh mushrooms.

1. Preheat oven to 400°F. In large, heavy ovenproof skillet, cook the bacon over medium heat until crisp, about 5 minutes, turning as needed. Drain on paper towels and set aside. In a large mixing bowl, combine the beef, Worcestershire, egg, egg white, salt, pepper, garlic powder, and onion. Mix well. Form into 4 patties.

2. Heat the skillet used to cook the bacon on medium-high, retaining about 1 tablespoon of the bacon grease in the pan. Sear the patties for about 2 minutes on each side. Place the skillet in the oven. Cook for about 5 minutes or to the desired doneness.

3. Assemble the burgers, using ½ slice bacon for each.

SERVES 4	
Serving size	1 burger

CALORIES PER SERVING	
Original recipe	870
SYS recipe	254

NUTRITIONAL BREAKDOWN	
Fat	9g
Carbohydrates	19g
Protein	28g
Sodium	353mg

swiss-me-miss-me mushroom burger

This recipe is filled with delicious and healthy substitutions such as lean ground turkey for beef, egg whites for whole eggs, reduced-fat Swiss cheese for whole-fat cheese, and high-fiber whole-grain buns instead of white-flour alternatives.

1 tablespoon butter

1½ cups sliced cremini mushrooms

1 white or yellow onion, halved and thinly sliced

Sea salt to taste

Black pepper to taste

¾ pound lean ground turkey

2 egg whites

1 teaspoon Italian seasoning

½ teaspoon garlic powder

4 slices reduced-fat Swiss cheese

4 whole-grain hamburger buns

Skinny Secret

If you would like to add mayonnaise, use ½ tablespoon of nonfat mayonnaise on each bun half, which adds only an additional 5 calories.

1. Preheat oven to 400°F. In a large ovenproof skillet, melt the butter over medium-low heat. Add the mushrooms and onions, and season with salt and pepper. Sauté until the onions are tender and slightly browned. Transfer to a bowl and set aside.

2. In a medium mixing bowl, combine the turkey, egg whites, seasoning, and garlic powder. Mix well. Form into 4 patties. Return the skillet to the stovetop (do not wipe out the skillet). Cook the patties until browned, about 2 minutes per side. Transfer the skillet to the oven and bake until the patties are cooked through, about 5 minutes. Top each patty with mushroom mixture, then top with cheese. Bake until the cheese is melted.

3. Assemble the burgers and enjoy!

SERVES 4		CALORIES PER SERVING		NUTRITIONAL BREAKDOWN	
Serving size	1 burger	Original recipe	542	Fat	20g
		SYS recipe	422	Carbohydrates	21g
				Protein	37g
				Sodium	347mg

gouda burger

Substitutions in this recipe make all the difference. With all the calories and fat you save by using a portobello mushroom as your "bun" and using lean ground turkey instead of higher-fat beef, you can afford the few extra calories in the Gouda cheese. For extra flavor, use smoked Gouda!

4 portobello mushrooms
1 tablespoon olive oil
¾ pound lean ground turkey
½ tablespoon minced fresh garlic
½ teaspoon sea salt
½ teaspoon black pepper
2 egg whites
¼ teaspoon ground mustard
1 teaspoon Worcestershire sauce
8 tablespoons diced Gouda cheese
Nonstick cooking spray

1. Preheat broiler. Place the mushrooms on a broiler pan and drizzle with olive oil. Broil until just tender, about 3 minutes. Remove from broiler and set aside. Preheat oven to 400°F.

2. In mixing bowl, mix together the turkey, garlic, salt, pepper, egg whites, mustard, and Worcestershire. Form into 4 patties. Spray a heavy ovenproof skillet with nonstick spray and heat on medium-high. Add the patties and sear for 2 minutes on each side to brown. Transfer the skillet to the oven and cook the patties until done, about 5 minutes. Top the patties with the cheese and return to the oven. Cook until the cheese melts, about 1 minute.

3. To serve, place each portobello mushroom, top side down, on a serving dish. Top each with a Gouda turkey burger and enjoy.

SERVES 4	
Serving size	1 patty with 2 tablespoons cheese

CALORIES PER SERVING	
Original recipe	630
SYS recipe	359

NUTRITIONAL BREAKDOWN	
Fat	23g
Carbohydrates	6g
Protein	33g
Sodium	503mg

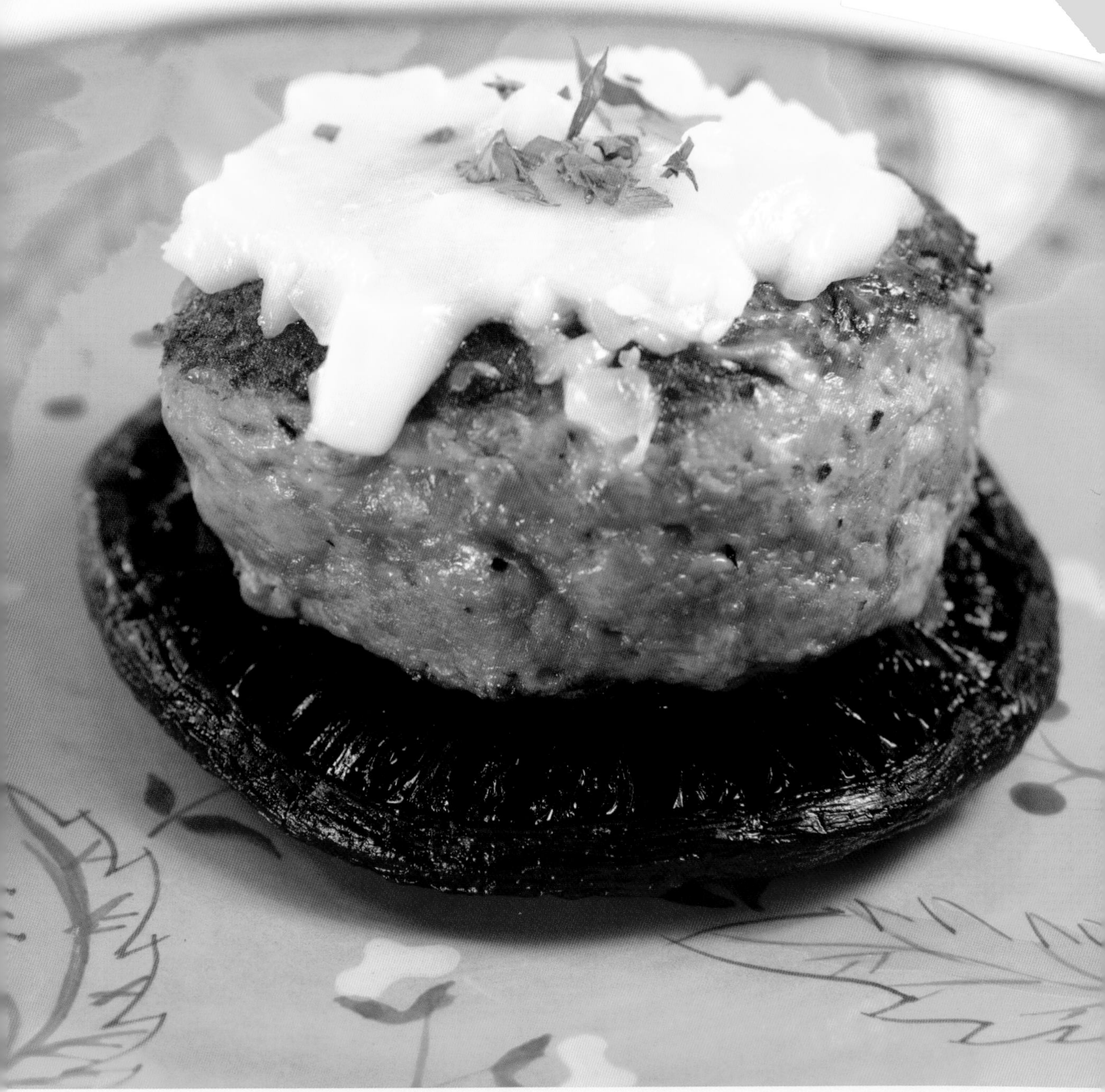

inch-away chicken enchilada

Skinless chicken breasts are naturally lean; however, make this dish even more slimming by substituting nonfat yogurt, reduced-fat cheese, reduced-fat tortillas, and nonstick cooking spray.

1 tablespoon butter

½ white or yellow onion, chopped

2 cups low-sodium chicken broth

1 cup plain nonfat yogurt

2 tablespoons pimento

1 tablespoon chili powder

1 (4-ounce) can green diced chilies

1 cup diced cooked chicken breast

¾ cup shredded reduced-fat Cheddar cheese

8 (6-inch) reduced-fat corn or flour tortillas

Nonstick cooking spray

Skinny Secret

Spice up this dish by adding sliced jalapeños and fresh tomatoes on the top after baking.

1. Preheat oven to 350°F. Spray a 9" × 9" baking dish with nonstick spray. In a large saucepan, melt the butter over medium heat. Add the onion and sauté until tender, about 5 minutes. Stir in the broth and then whisk in the yogurt until combined. Whisk in the pimento, chili powder, and chilies until combined. Cover, reduce heat, and simmer for about 20 minutes, stirring occasionally. Ladle 1 cup of sauce in a mixing bowl and add the chicken. Stir to coat.

2. Dip a tortilla in the sauce, then place it in the prepared baking dish. Spoon 2 tablespoons of the chicken mixture onto the tortilla, and top with 1 tablespoon of cheese. Roll up the tortilla. Repeat with the remaining tortillas. Pour the remaining sauce on top of the enchiladas and top with the remaining cheese. Bake for 30 minutes, and serve.

SERVES 8		CALORIES PER SERVING		NUTRITIONAL BREAKDOWN	
Serving size	1 enchilada	Original recipe	530	Fat	8g
		SYS recipe	217	Carbohydrates	22g
				Protein	15g
				Sodium	488mg

cinch-an-inch beef enchilada

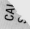

Substituting in this recipe is made simple by using 95 percent lean ground beef; reduced-fat cheese; reduced-calorie, higher-fiber corn tortillas; and nonstick cooking spray instead of oil or butter.

Nonstick cooking spray

For the sauce:

½ pound 95 percent lean ground beef

½ white or yellow onion, chopped

1 clove garlic, chopped

½ cup low-sodium, fat-free chicken broth

2 cans tomato paste

2 teaspoons chili powder

1 teaspoon ground cumin

Sea salt to taste

Black pepper to taste

For the enchiladas:

Nonstick cooking spray

1 tablespoon olive oil

½ white or yellow onion, chopped

1 (10-ounce) can green chilies

8 small reduced-calorie corn tortillas

¼ cup chopped pitted black olives

1 cup shredded reduced-fat Monterey jack cheese

1. Preheat oven to 350°F. Spray an 8-inch rectangular baking dish with nonstick spray. Make the sauce: Heat a heavy skillet on medium. Add the beef, onions, and garlic. Sauté until the beef is browned and the onion is tender, about 7 minutes. Add the broth, paste, chili powder, and cumin. Stir to combine.

2. Reduce heat to low, cover, and simmer for about 20 minutes. Season with salt and pepper, stir, cover, and simmer for an additional 10 minutes. Set aside.

3. Make the enchiladas: Heat the oil in a heavy skillet over medium heat. Add the onion and sauté for about 4 minutes, just until tender. Add the chilies and sauté until heated through, about 1½ minutes. Turn off heat. Heat the tortillas in the microwave for about 15 seconds. Do not overheat. Dip 1 tortilla in the sauce mixture and place in the prepared baking dish. Fill with 1 to 1½ tablespoons onion mixture, top with ½ tablespoon olives and 1 tablespoon cheese, and roll up. Repeat with the remaining tortillas. Top the enchiladas with the remaining sauce and any remaining cheese and olives.

4. Bake for 20 minutes. Serve 1 enchilada per person.

SERVES 8		CALORIES PER SERVING		NUTRITIONAL BREAKDOWN	
Serving size	1 enchilada	Original recipe	568	Fat	11g
		SYS recipe	280	Carbohydrates	28g
				Protein	19g
				Sodium	670mg

feelin' saucy spaghetti with sausage

Low-fat turkey sausage makes all the difference in this recipe. Whole-wheat spaghetti provides needed fiber that helps break down proteins.

½ pound low-fat turkey sausage, removed from casing
1 yellow onion, chopped
1 (28- or 29-ounce) can tomato sauce
1 (14.5-ounce) can diced tomatoes
1 bay leaf
1 teaspoon dried Italian seasoning
½ teaspoon garlic powder
½ tablespoon chopped fresh basil leaves
1 teaspoon chopped fresh oregano leaves
Sea salt to taste
Black pepper to taste
8 ounces dried whole-wheat spaghetti

Skinny Secret

For an even leaner pasta, omit the sausage and add veggies such as broccoli and red bell peppers.

1. In a large skillet over medium heat, cook the sausage and onion until the sausage is browned, about 6 minutes, breaking up the sausage as it cooks. Add the tomato sauce, tomatoes, bay leaf, seasoning, garlic powder, basil, oregano, and salt and pepper. Mix well, reduce heat to low, and cover. Simmer for about 30 minutes, adding water if needed to thin out the sauce.

2. Bring a large pot of water to a boil. Add the pasta, and cook until al dente, about 8 to 10 minutes. Drain well. Add the sauce and toss well.

3. Serve in 1-cup portions on dinner plates.

SERVES 8		CALORIES PER SERVING		NUTRITIONAL BREAKDOWN	
Serving size	1 cup	Original recipe	601	Fat	2g
		SYS recipe	251	Carbohydrates	28g
				Protein	14g
				Sodium	713mg

crazy chicken

Many Jamaican jerk chicken recipes call for sugar. Skip the sugar and substitute fresh lime juice and orange juice. Marinating for several hours in the refrigerator gives all the flavor you need.

1 white or yellow onion, chopped

2 cloves garlic, chopped

1 jalapeño, seeded and chopped

2 teaspoons allspice

2 teaspoons black pepper

1 teaspoon nutmeg

½ teaspoon cinnamon

1 tablespoon chopped fresh thyme leaves

2 teaspoons sea salt

1 tablespoon canola oil

1 tablespoon honey

Juice of 1 orange

Juice of 3 limes

3 tablespoons low-sodium soy sauce

1 (3-pound) whole chicken, cut up into serving pieces, skin removed

Nonstick cooking spray

1. In a food processor, combine all the ingredients except the chicken, and purée into a paste. Spread the paste all over the chicken. Place the chicken in large sealable bags and refrigerate for 4 hours or overnight.

2. When ready to bake, preheat oven to 400°F. Spray a large baking dish with nonstick spray. Place the chicken in the dish and bake for 45 minutes, until cooked through and browned. Serve 1 piece per person.

Skinny Secret

Add even more flavor to this dish without adding calories by adding freshly diced tomatoes and 1 tablespoon of fresh cilantro to the onion mixture while cooking.

SERVES 6		CALORIES PER SERVING		NUTRITIONAL BREAKDOWN	
Serving size	1 piece of chicken	Original recipe	336	Fat	14g
		SYS recipe	205	Carbohydrates	6g
				Protein	14g
				Sodium	351mg

slimmy chimmy-changas

Keep these chimichangas slimming by substituting skinless chicken breasts, low-carb tortillas, fat-free refried beans, reduced-fat cheese, and nonfat sour cream.

1 tablespoon taco seasoning

2 tablespoons green chilies, chopped

2 tablespoons mild or hot salsa

4 tablespoons diced cooked chicken breast

2 (10-inch) reduced-fat low-carb flour tortillas

4 tablespoons fat-free refried beans

4 tablespoons shredded reduced-fat Cheddar cheese

2 tablespoons shredded reduced-fat Monterey jack cheese

2 tablespoons nonfat sour cream

Nonstick cooking spray

Skinny Secret

These make large servings. Split in half and make 4 servings for an even leaner meal without sacrificing flavor. Serve with a light side salad such as Wow, That's a Caesar Salad (recipe, page 38).

1. Preheat oven to 375°F. Spray a small baking dish with nonstick cooking spray. In a mixing bowl, combine the taco seasoning, green chilies, salsa, and chicken. Mix well. Lay the tortillas on a flat work surface, spread 2 tablespoons of the refried beans on top of each, and divide the chicken mixture between the tortillas. Top each with 2 tablespoons Cheddar cheese, 1 tablespoon jack cheese, and 1 tablespoon sour cream. Fold in sides and roll tortilla, creating a "loaf." Place the chimichangas in the prepared baking dish (or you can bake them on a baking sheet sprayed with nonstick spray or lined with parchment paper).

2. Bake the chimichangas for about 30 minutes. Serve 1 chimichanga per person with additional salsa, if desired.

SERVES 2	
Serving size	1 chimichanga

CALORIES PER SERVING	
Original recipe	441
SYS recipe	381

NUTRITIONAL BREAKDOWN	
Fat	12g
Carbohydrates	52g
Protein	27g
Sodium	1,472mg

bavarian cornish hens

CALORIE SAVINGS

118

Lean turkey sausage is used to stuff these hens, saving more than 25 calories per serving compared to regular sausage. For an even healthier meal full of fiber, use cooked brown rice instead of white rice.

4 ounces lean turkey sausage

¼ cup diced Golden Delicious apples

¼ cup diced celery

⅓ cup diced white or yellow onion

3 tablespoons low-sodium chicken broth

Juice of ½ lemon

1 tablespoon chopped fresh sage leaves

2 cups cooked white rice

Sea salt to taste

Black pepper to taste

2 Cornish game hens, rinsed

1. Preheat oven to 400°F. Prepare a medium roasting pan by spraying with nonstick spray. In a heavy skillet, brown the sausage over medium heat. Add the apples, celery, and onion. Sauté until all are tender, about 5 minutes. Add the chicken broth, lemon juice, and sage. Stir to combine. Add the rice and mix well.

2. Stuff each hen with ¼ to ½ cup of rice mixture. Season the outside of the hens lightly with salt and pepper. Transfer to the prepared baking dish and bake, uncovered, for about 1 hour. If the hens begin to brown too dark on top, cover loosely with foil for the last 15 minutes of baking time. Serve ½ hen per person.

Skinny Secret

Cornish hens are a great way to have a nutritious meal all in one. Other healthy ingredients you could add to this recipe are chopped broccoli florets, red bell peppers, or corn. If adding, use about ¼ cup and add with the apples.

SERVES 4		CALORIES PER SERVING		NUTRITIONAL BREAKDOWN	
Serving size	½ stuffed hen	Original recipe	510	Fat	20g
		SYS recipe	392	Carbohydrates	25g
				Protein	32g
				Sodium	101mg

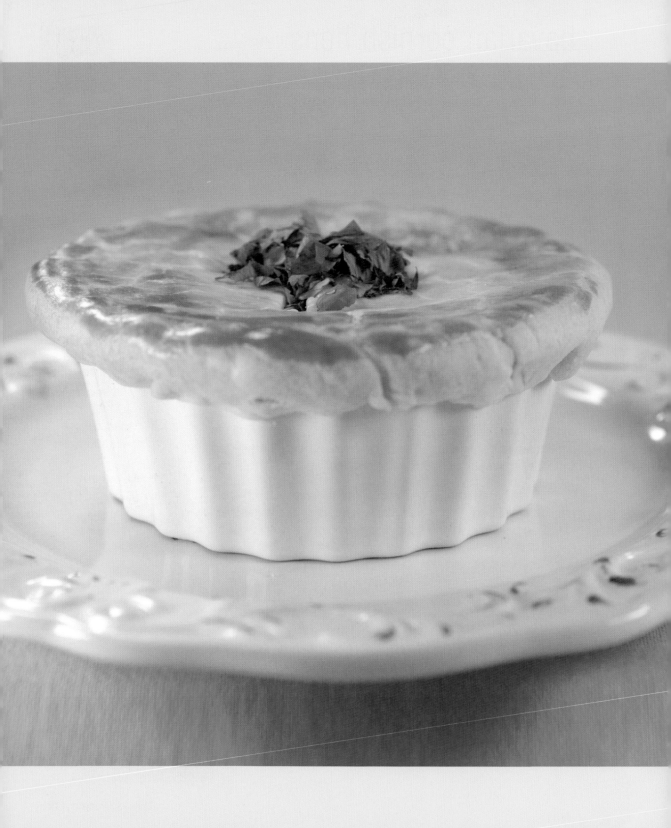

no pot belly here
chicken potpie

Leaving off the bottom crust of the potpie saves over 250 calories per recipe! If you don't have a 5-inch round pastry cutter, place a 5-inch round bowl face-down on pastry and use a butter knife to cut out dough.

Nonstick cooking spray
4 (4-ounce) boneless, skinless chicken breasts
Sea salt to taste
Black pepper to taste
½ cup water
1 (10¾-ounce) can reduced-fat condensed cream of mushroom soup
1 pound frozen mixed vegetables
1 package (contains 2) 9-inch pie crust dough

1. Preheat oven to 375°F. Spray the ramekins with nonstick spray. Season the chicken breasts with salt and pepper. Add the chicken and water to a large skillet and heat on medium. Cover, reduce heat to medium-low, and cook until done, about 15 to 18 minutes. Transfer the chicken to a cutting board and dice. Return the chicken to the pan and add the mushroom soup and vegetables. Season to taste with salt and pepper. Let simmer for 12 minutes. Ladle ½ cup chicken mixture into each ramekin.

2. For the topping, roll out a pie crust. Using a 5-inch round pastry cutter, cut a circle out large enough to cover the tops of the ramekins. Place circle of dough on top of each ramekin and pinch it down around the edges.

3. Bake for 45 minutes or until the crust is golden and the center is heated through. Serve 1 potpie per person.

SERVES 8		CALORIES PER SERVING		NUTRITIONAL BREAKDOWN	
Serving size	1 pie	Original recipe	520	Fat	10g
		SYS recipe	266	Carbohydrates	21g
				Protein	21g
				Sodium	366mg

creamy clam chowder

Clam chowder doesn't have to be fattening. Substitute lean turkey bacon, reduce the amount of butter used, and use nonfat milk for a truly creamy chowder that's good for your figure.

3 (8-ounce) bottles clam juice
2 large baking potatoes, peeled and cut into ½-inch pieces
1 slice turkey bacon, diced
1 large white or yellow onion, diced
1¼ cup diced celery
2 garlic cloves, minced
1 tablespoon butter
¼ cup plain flour
1 (15-ounce) can kernel corn, drained
1¼ cups nonfat milk
2 dashes hot sauce
6 (6.5-ounce) cans chopped clams, juice reserved
Sea salt to taste
Black pepper to taste

Skinny Secret

For a less chunky, more creamy chowder, purée the potatoes, with liquid, in batches and then add as directed to recipe. This recipe freezes well; freeze in individual containers for up to 2 months.

1. In large-quart boiler, combine the clam juice and potatoes. Bring to a boil over medium heat and cook until the potatoes are tender, about 15 minutes. Do not drain. In another large-quart boiler, sauté the bacon, onion, celery, and garlic over medium heat until the bacon is soft, but cooked, and the onion is tender. Add the butter, and stir until melted. Stir in the flour until a thick paste forms. Whisk in the corn, milk, and hot sauce; stir until well blended. Add the potatoes with the liquid, and the clams with the juice, and stir. Cover and simmer over low heat for 20 minutes, stirring occasionally, adding salt and pepper to taste.

2. To serve, ladle 1-cup portions into bowls for an entrée, or ½-cup servings for a side dish.

SERVES 6		CALORIES PER SERVING		NUTRITIONAL BREAKDOWN	
Serving size	1 cup	Original recipe	522	Fat	7g
		SYS recipe	433	Carbohydrates	38g
				Protein	53g
				Sodium	406mg

lovin' linguine with clams

The key substitution here is whole-wheat pasta, which is high in fiber, lower in calories, and full of flavor. Other ways this recipe is made lean is by using less olive oil, low-sodium chicken broth, and passing on the cheese.

8 ounces dried whole-wheat linguine pasta

1 tablespoon olive oil

1 shallot, chopped

1 clove garlic, chopped

1 Roma tomato, seeded and diced

Juice of 1 lemon, then slice the lemon into ¼-inch slices

1 cup dry white wine such as sauvignon blanc

1 cup low-sodium chicken broth

2 tablespoons fresh Italian flat-leaf parsley

2 dozen littleneck clams, scrubbed

White pepper to taste

1. Prepare the pasta as directed on the package. In a large saucepan, heat the oil on medium and add the shallot and garlic. Sauté until tender, about 4 minutes. Add the tomatoes and cook for 1 minute. Add the lemon juice and wine. Stir and cook for 1 to 2 minutes. Add the broth and parsley. Bring to a boil, then reduce heat and simmer for 5 minutes. Add the clams, cover, and cook until all are opened, discarding any that do not open.

2. Transfer the clams to a separate bowl. Return the mixture to a boil and boil until reduced by ⅓. Meanwhile, remove the clams from the shells. Toss the pasta with the sauce. Divide between 4 serving dishes, about 1 cup each. Add the clams, distributed equally among the 4 servings, about 3 clams each. Garnish with sliced lemons, if desired.

Skinny Secret

Clams are remarkably high in protein, with 14 grams per dozen, and very low in fat, with less than 1 gram of fat per dozen.

SERVES 4		CALORIES PER SERVING		NUTRITIONAL BREAKDOWN	
Serving size	1 cup pasta with ¼ cup sauce	Original recipe	567	Fat	5g
		SYS recipe	325	Carbohydrates	46g
				Protein	14g
				Sodium	48mg

creamy salmon pasta

Broiling salmon is a lean, healthy way to prepare this fish, which is high in the natural good fats your body needs. Keep this dish even leaner by making your cream sauce with nonfat milk and nonfat sour cream as opposed to using high-fat heavy whipping cream.

8 ounces penne pasta
½ pound salmon fillet
Sea salt to taste
Black pepper to taste
1 tablespoon olive oil
1 shallot, minced
1 teaspoon Dijon mustard
½ tablespoon chopped fresh tarragon leaves
2 tablespoons plain flour
½ cup nonfat milk
½ cup nonfat sour cream
2 tablespoons grated Parmesan cheese

Skinny Secret

Salmon is very healthy because it is high in omega-3 fatty acids, which are great for your skin and naturally low in calories.

1. Preheat broiler. Prepare the pasta as directed on the package. Place the salmon on aluminum foil and season lightly with salt and pepper. Place under the broiler for about 5 minutes. Remove from heat and set aside.

2. In a large saucepan, heat the oil on medium and add the shallots. Sauté until tender, about 3 minutes. Add the mustard and tarragon; sauté for 1 minute. Add the flour and stir into a paste. Whisk in the milk and sour cream. Cook until heated through, stirring often. Add the salmon and break into pieces. Toss with the pasta and serve in 4 equal portions.

SERVES 4

Serving size	1 cup

CALORIES PER SERVING

Original recipe	500
SYS recipe	382

NUTRITIONAL BREAKDOWN

Fat	9g
Carbohydrates	52g
Protein	23g
Sodium	129mg

veggie risotto

Traditional risotto dishes often use lots and lots of cheese. This recipe focuses on the high-flavor, colorful vegetables, uses low-sodium, fat-free chicken broth, and keeps cheese to a minimum.

1 tablespoon olive oil

2 garlic cloves, chopped

½ white or yellow onion, chopped

Fine zest of 1 lemon

½ cup white wine such as sauvignon blanc

½ cup chopped broccoli florets

1 red bell pepper, seeded and diced

1 yellow summer squash, diced

1½ cups arborio rice

5 cups low-sodium, fat-free chicken broth, brought to a boil and simmering

2 tablespoons grated Parmesan cheese

Sea salt to taste

Black pepper to taste

1. In a large-quart boiler, heat the olive oil over medium heat. Add the garlic, onion, and lemon. Sauté until the onion is tender, about 4 minutes. Add the white wine, broccoli, bell pepper, and squash; sauté for about 1 minute. Add the rice and stir to brown, about 2 minutes. Add ½ cup of the hot chicken broth to the rice mixture. Cook, stirring frequently, until all the moisture has been absorbed.

2. Continue adding the broth in ½ cup increments until all the broth has been added. Once all broth has been added, cook until the rice is soft but still slightly al dente. Stir in the cheese and season with salt and pepper. Serve in ¾-cup portions.

Skinny Secret

This recipe only uses fresh vegetables and no fish or other proteins, so you can afford the few calories in the Parmesan cheese.

SERVES 4	
Serving size	¾ cup

CALORIES PER SERVING	
Original recipe	330
SYS recipe	217

NUTRITIONAL BREAKDOWN	
Fat	11g
Carbohydrates	11g
Protein	14g
Sodium	69mg

rock 'n' roll shrimp risotto

Risotto sometimes gets a bad rap, but it's usually because of all the cheese. Skip the cheese but maximize the flavor with fresh asparagus and lemon.

1 tablespoon olive oil

½ white or yellow onion, chopped

2 garlic cloves, chopped

Fine zest of 1 lemon

½ cup white wine such as sauvignon blanc

½ cup chopped asparagus tips

1½ cups arborio rice

5 cups low-sodium chicken broth, brought to a boil and simmering

½ pound cooked medium shrimp, peeled and deveined

Sea salt to taste

Black pepper to taste

Skinny Secret

Seafood, in general, is low in fat and calories. This recipe is equally delicious substituted with scallops.

1. In a large-quart boiler, heat the olive oil on medium. Add the onion, garlic, and lemon zest. Sauté until the onion is tender, about 4 minutes. Add the wine and asparagus tips. Cook about 1 minute. Add the rice and stir to brown, about 2 minutes. Add ½ cup of the hot chicken broth to the rice mixture. Cook, stirring frequently, until the moisture has been absorbed.

2. Continue adding the broth ½ cup at a time until all the broth has been added. Once all the broth has been added, cook until the rice is soft but still slightly al dente. Add the shrimp, season with salt and pepper, and serve in ¾-cup portions.

SERVES 4		CALORIES PER SERVING		NUTRITIONAL BREAKDOWN	
Serving size	¾ cup	Original recipe	620	Fat	2g
		SYS recipe	238	Carbohydrates	30g
				Protein	23g
				Sodium	131mg

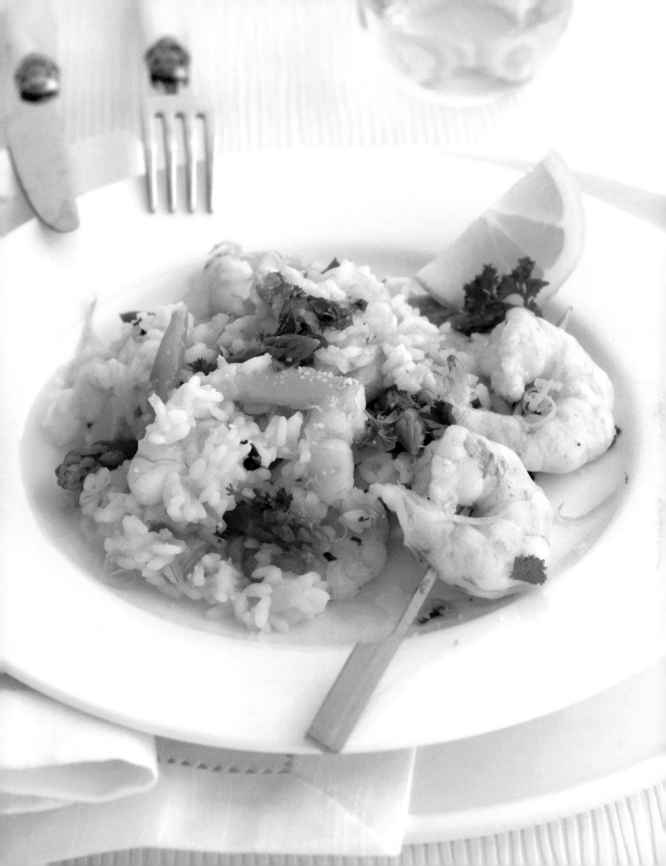

no-dimple dumplings with chicken

Using reduced-fat Bisquick saves 60 calories per recipe.
Old-fashioned dumplings are made with lard!

2 cups reduced-fat Bisquick baking mix
2 (10¾-ounce) cans fat-free condensed cream of chicken soup
2 boneless, skinless chicken breasts, chopped
2 carrots, peeled and chopped
1 white or yellow onion, chopped
2 celery stalks, chopped
1 (14-ounce) can low-sodium, fat-free chicken broth
Sea salt to taste
Black pepper to taste
1 cup water

1. Prepare the dumplings as directed on the package, using water.
Heat a large-quart boiler on medium heat. Add the soup and chicken.
Cook until the chicken is cooked through, about 8 minutes.

2. Add the carrots, onion, celery, and broth. Stir well to combine.
Bring to a boil and cook for 20 minutes. Season with salt and pepper
as desired. Add the water and return to a boil. Add the dumplings
and cook until they rise to the top.

3. Serve 2 dumplings per person with 1 cup soup.

SERVES 4	
Serving size	1 cup

CALORIES PER SERVING	
Original recipe	504
SYS recipe	402

NUTRITIONAL BREAKDOWN	
Fat	9g
Carbohydrates	54g
Protein	24g
Sodium	1,316mg

chicken cordon bleu

CALORIE SAVINGS
203

This dish is made lean with lean turkey ham, reduced-fat mozzarella cheese, nonfat milk, fat-free cream of celery soup, and nonfat sour cream. Enjoying the chicken without the skin also cuts out calories.

4 boneless, skinless chicken breasts, about 4 ounces each
½ teaspoon black pepper
4 ounces lean deli turkey ham
½ cup reduced-fat shredded mozzarella cheese
⅓ cup nonfat milk
½ cup crushed puffed rice cereal
1 teaspoon paprika
½ teaspoon garlic powder
¼ teaspoon sea salt
½ (10¾-ounce) can fat-free condensed cream of celery soup
¼ cup nonfat sour cream
1 tablespoon chopped fresh Italian parsley leaves
Fine zest of ½ lemon
Juice of ½ lemon

1. Place the chicken on a cutting board, cover with wax paper, and pound with a meat pounder until ¼ inch thick. Season with pepper. Top each with ham and place 2 tablespoons of mozzarella cheese down the center of the ham. Roll up and secure with toothpicks.

2. Preheat oven to 350°F. Spray an 8-inch square baking dish with nonstick spray. Pour milk into a shallow bowl. In separate bowl, combine the cereal, paprika, garlic powder, and salt. Dip the chicken in the milk, then roll in the cereal. Place in the prepared baking dish. Bake, uncovered, for 25 to 30 minutes or until cooked through.

3. While the chicken is baking, combine the soup, sour cream, parsley, lemon zest, and juice in a small saucepan over medium heat. Stir to mix well, and cook until heated through. Serve 1 chicken breast with 2 tablespoons of sauce.

Skinny Secret

This recipe makes a great healthy appetizer. To serve as an appetizer, simply cut the cooked chicken "rolls" into ¼- to ½-inch slices and top with 1 teaspoon of sauce.

SERVES 4	
Serving size	1 piece of chicken

CALORIES PER SERVING	
Original recipe	509
SYS recipe	306

NUTRITIONAL BREAKDOWN	
Fat	8g
Carbohydrates	13g
Protein	43g
Sodium	439mg

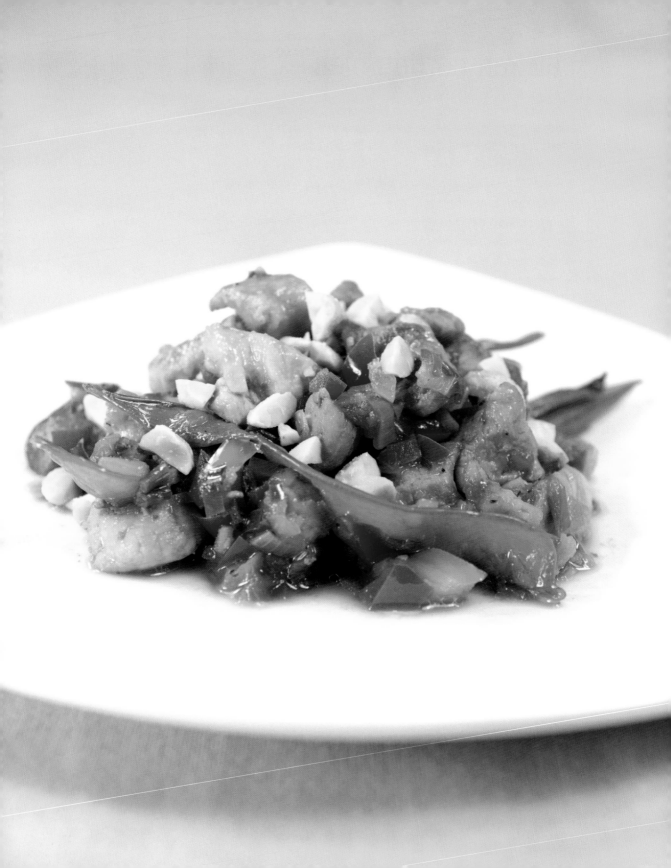

kung-pow pork

Trimming the fat off any meat keeps fat out without sacrificing flavor and is evidenced here with this fat-trimmed lean pork. Cutting back on the amount of peanuts keeps fat and calories to a minimum but still gives this dish that delicious nutty flavor.

1 tablespoon canola oil
¾ pound pork loin, trimmed of fat and cut into 1-inch cubes
1 clove garlic, minced
Fine zest of 1 orange
1½ tablespoons sherry wine
4 dried chili peppers, minced
½ red bell pepper, chopped
½ yellow bell pepper, chopped
1 cup snow peas, left whole
4 green onions, green and white parts, minced
2 tablespoons low-sodium soy sauce
½ tablespoon minced fresh gingerroot
1 tablespoon honey
1 tablespoon chopped roasted peanuts

1. In a large saucepan, heat the oil on medium and add the pork. Cook until just cooked through, about 3 minutes. Add the garlic and orange zest. Cook for about 1 minute. Add the sherry, chili peppers, bell peppers, snow peas, onions, soy sauce, gingerroot, and honey. Sauté for about 3 to 4 minutes.

2. When the vegetables are just tender, add the peanuts. Serve on plates in 1-cup portions.

Skinny Secret

Usually Asian dishes such as this one are served with steamed rice. Serve this over lettuce-leaf cups instead for a truly lean dish.

SERVES 4			CALORIES PER SERVING		NUTRITIONAL BREAKDOWN	
Serving size	1 cup		Original recipe	500	Fat	19g
			SYS recipe	275	Carbohydrates	9g
					Protein	26g
					Sodium	421mg

dijon pork

Usually, Dijon pork chops are breaded using a milk-and-egg mixture and seasoned bread crumbs; the chops are then fried in oil. Maximize the mustard flavor without adding the carbs by searing and then baking the chops in the oven.

3 tablespoons Dijon mustard
2 tablespoons nonfat mayonnaise
4 (4-ounce) bone-in pork chops
Sea salt to taste
Black pepper to taste
Nonstick cooking spray

Skinny Secret

Pork pairs well with lots of flavors, including sweet citrus, spicy, and sour (such as vinegar). Pork is actually lower in calories than both chicken and turkey.

1. Preheat oven to 400°F. In a small bowl, combine the mustard and mayonnaise. Season the pork chops lightly with salt and pepper. Smear each chop with the mustard mixture on both sides. Spray an ovenproof skillet with nonstick spray and heat on medium. Add the pork chops and sear on each side, about 3 minutes each.

2. Transfer the skillet to the oven and finish cooking the chops, about 3 minutes, or until done. Serve 1 chop per person.

SERVES 4	
Serving size	1 chop

CALORIES PER SERVING	
Original recipe	270
SYS recipe	213

NUTRITIONAL BREAKDOWN	
Fat	11g
Carbohydrates	1g
Protein	23g
Sodium	370mg

slimming sides

not-so-scalloped potatoes

Scalloped potatoes can be very fattening, since they are usually prepared with whole milk and often, lots of cheese. This recipe cuts down the calories by using nonfat milk, minimal amounts of flour, and skipping the cheese. If you absolutely must have cheese, use ¼ cup reduced-fat white Cheddar and add it after you add the milk mixture, just before you toss the potatoes.

Nonstick cooking spray
4 large red potatoes, peeled and cut into ¼-inch slices
1 tablespoon olive oil
1 large shallot, peeled and diced
2 tablespoons plain flour
1¾ cups nonfat milk
1 teaspoon sea salt
1 teaspoon ground black pepper
½ teaspoon dry mustard
Small pinch ground nutmeg

1. Preheat oven to 350°F. Prepare a small rectangular baking dish by spraying with nonstick spray. Place the potatoes in a large mixing bowl and set aside.

2. In a heavy saucepan, heat the oil on medium for a few seconds. Add the shallots and sauté until tender, about 3 minutes. Add the flour and stir to combine. Add the milk, salt, and pepper and cook until just bubbling. Add the mustard and nutmeg, and stir. Pour the milk mixture over the potatoes and toss to coat.

3. Transfer to the prepared baking dish, cover with aluminum foil, and bake for 30 to 40 minutes. Uncover and bake for an additional 10 to 15 minutes or until the potatoes are tender.

Skinny Secret

When eating super-rich dishes like this one, it is easy to consume a large portion in a very short amount of time. The key is to place your serving on a plate and then enjoy each bite, one by one . . . dissecting the flavors and textures slowly in your mouth. Allowing yourself to enjoy the food helps prevent overeating in two ways: one, you actually enjoy the food more; and two, you allow your body to communicate with your brain that it is satisfied.

SERVES 4	
Serving size	½ cup

CALORIES PER SERVING	
Original recipe	378
SYS recipe	232

NUTRITIONAL BREAKDOWN	
Fat	4g
Carbohydrates	35g
Protein	6g
Sodium	44mg

oh-so-creamy creamed corn

Creamed corn is a favorite side dish that doesn't have to be overly fattening when you substitute nonfat sweetened condensed milk for its high-fat counterpart. Cutting back on sugar and using nonfat milk are also key thinning tips.

10 ounces frozen kernel corn

¾ cup nonfat sweetened condensed milk

Pinch sea salt

1 tablespoon granulated sugar

Pinch ground black pepper

1 tablespoon unsalted butter

¾ cup nonfat milk

1 tablespoon plain flour

1½ tablespoons grated Parmesan cheese (optional)

In a heavy skillet over medium heat, combine the corn, condensed milk, salt, sugar, pepper, and butter. Whisk together the milk and flour and stir into the corn mixture. Cook over medium heat, stirring constantly, until the mixture is thickened and the corn is cooked through. Remove from heat, stir in the Parmesan cheese, and serve hot.

Skinny Secret

Eating at home helps you control the calories and nutrients you consume. Try making simple recipes like this one to become more at ease with your cooking skills, which will encourage you to cook at home.

SERVES 6		CALORIES PER SERVING		NUTRITIONAL BREAKDOWN	
Serving size	½ cup	Original recipe	257	Fat	3g
		SYS recipe	177	Carbohydrates	13g
				Protein	4g
				Sodium	312mg

floren-lean potatoes

Traditional Florentine dishes are made with heavy cream sauces and spinach. Keep the spinach in but fat out by cutting back on the amount of butter used and substituting nonfat milk and reduced-fat blue cheese.

½ tablespoon olive oil

2 cups chopped fresh spinach leaves

1 shallot, minced

3 large baking potatoes, peeled and cut into 1-inch cubes

1 cup nonfat milk

2 tablespoons butter

¼ cup reduced-fat blue cheese crumbles

Sea salt to taste

Black pepper to taste

Skinny Secret

If you can live without it, skip the cheese and save 80 calories and 5 grams of fat per recipe.

1. In a medium saucepan, heat the olive oil on medium. Add the spinach and shallots. Stir until wilted, about 3 minutes. In a large-quart boiler, add the potatoes and fill the boiler with enough water to cover the potatoes. Bring to a boil and cook until the potatoes are tender, about 20 minutes. Drain well.

2. Return the potatoes to the pan, and add the milk, butter and cheese. Mash with a potato masher until well combined. Season to taste with salt and pepper. Stir in spinach mixture until well combined. Serve hot in ½-cup servings.

SERVES 6	
Serving size	½ cup

CALORIES PER SERVING	
Original recipe	453
SYS recipe	166

NUTRITIONAL BREAKDOWN	
Fat	7g
Carbohydrates	21g
Protein	6g
Sodium	117mg

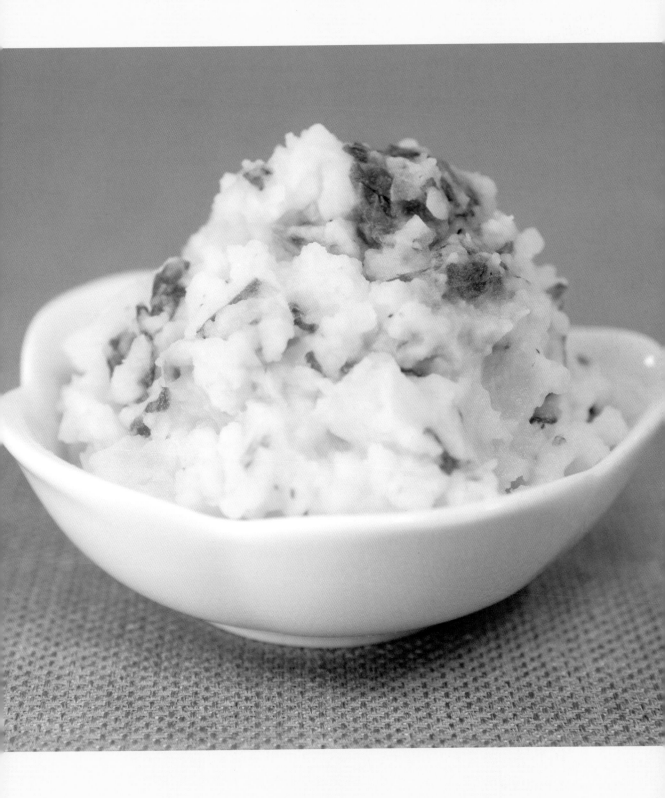

creamiest creamed spinach

Traditional creamed spinach is full of heavy cream and butter, which will go straight to your hips! Keep the calories off your waistline by using nonfat milk and sour cream.

¼ cup water
3 (10-ounce) bags fresh spinach, washed, dried, and chopped
1 tablespoon butter
2 cloves garlic, minced
½ white onion, chopped
1 cup nonfat milk
½ cup nonfat sour cream
½ cup reduced-fat mozzarella cheese
¼ cup grated Parmesan cheese
Sea salt to taste
White pepper to taste

1. In a large skillet, heat ¼ cup water on medium-low, and add the spinach. Cover, and cook until the spinach wilts, about 3 minutes. Remove from the skillet and drain.

2. Return the skillet to the stovetop, and increase heat to medium. Add the butter, garlic, and onion. Sauté until tender, about 4 minutes. Add the spinach and stir. Add the milk and sour cream, and stir until well blended. Add the mozzarella and Parmesan. Season with salt and pepper to taste.

3. Cook until the cheeses are melted and blended. Serve in ½-cup portions while hot.

Skinny Secret

Extra spice can temporarily increase your metabolism. Add a dash or two of cayenne pepper or hot sauce for a flavor kick with no added calories.

SERVES 10	
Serving size	½ cup

CALORIES PER SERVING	
Original recipe	248
SYS recipe	82

NUTRITIONAL BREAKDOWN	
Fat	4g
Carbohydrates	7g
Protein	9g
Sodium	111mg

cheesy green beans with water chestnuts

Traditional green bean casseroles usually use canned fried onion rings and heavy creamed soups. Omitting the fried onions and substituting a few bread crumbs saves more than 76 grams of fat!

1 (10¾-ounce) can fat-free condensed cream of celery soup
⅓ cup nonfat sour cream
¼ teaspoon black pepper
¼ teaspoon sea salt
Fine zest of ½ lemon
Juice of ½ lemon
2 cups fresh green beans, cut into 1-inch pieces
½ white onion, chopped
½ cup reduced-fat Swiss cheese
1 can sliced water chestnuts, drained

For the topping:

2 tablespoons butter, melted
¼ cup Italian-style bread crumbs
¼ cup grated Parmesan cheese

1. Preheat oven to 375°F. Spray a round or rectangular 2-quart casserole dish with nonstick spray. In a large mixing bowl, combine the soup, sour cream, pepper, salt, lemon zest and juice, beans, onions, Swiss cheese, and water chestnuts. Mix well. Pour into the prepared baking dish and bake for 40 minutes.

2. Meanwhile, in a small bowl, combine the butter, bread crumbs and Parmesan cheese. Remove the casserole from the oven, and sprinkle the Parmesan mixture on top. Return to the oven and finish baking for about 10 minutes, or until the crumbs begin to brown. Serve hot in ½-cup portions.

SERVES 10		CALORIES PER SERVING		NUTRITIONAL BREAKDOWN	
Serving size	½ cup	Original recipe	281	Fat	5g
		SYS recipe	96	Carbohydrates	8g
				Protein	4g
				Sodium	198mg

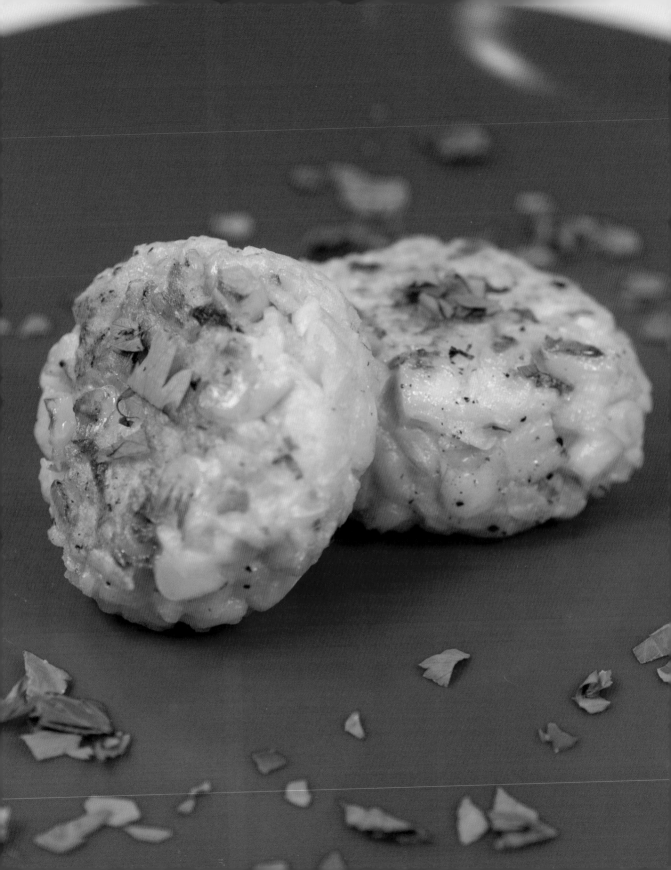

roastin' it corn and rice cakes

Substituting high-fiber, high-nutrient brown rice, lighter panko bread crumbs, and a leaner combination of 1 whole egg and 1 egg white instead of 2 whole eggs makes these tasty cakes not only deliciously slimming but good for you.

1 cup instant brown rice

2 tablespoons olive oil

3 green onions, chopped

1 clove garlic, minced

1 teaspoon chopped fresh thyme leaves

1 teaspoon chopped fresh cilantro leaves

Fine zest of 1 lemon

1 cup fresh frozen corn kernels

½ cup Japanese panko bread crumbs

½ teaspoon sea salt

½ teaspoon black pepper

1 egg

1 egg white

Skinny Secret

These mini cakes are a perfect appetizer or side dish and can be made ahead and frozen for up to 2 months.

1. Prepare the rice as directed on the package. Transfer to a large mixing bowl and mash with a potato masher or fork.

2. In a large saucepan, heat 1 tablespoon of the oil over medium heat. Add the onions, garlic, thyme, cilantro, lemon zest, and corn. Sauté for about 2 minutes. Transfer to the mixing bowl with the rice. Add the bread crumbs, salt, pepper, egg, and egg white. Mold into 8 small round cakes.

3. Heat the remaining olive oil in the same skillet over medium heat. Add the cakes and sauté until the outside is crisp and slightly browned, about 3 minutes per side. Serve hot.

SERVES 4	
Serving size	2 cakes

CALORIES PER SERVING	
Original recipe	275
SYS recipe	175

NUTRITIONAL BREAKDOWN	
Fat	10g
Carbohydrates	51g
Protein	10g
Sodium	52mg

grillin' 'n' chillin' asparagus with cheese

Substituting egg whites for whole eggs is an easy way to cut out calories, fat, and even cholesterol! Replacing whole-milk products with nonfat milk and nonfat sour cream gives you the creamy texture you love without those extra calories.

1½ cups chopped asparagus spears

2 eggs, beaten

3 egg whites, lightly beaten

1½ cups nonfat milk

1 cup nonfat sour cream

¼ cup grated Parmesan cheese

¼ cup Japanese panko bread crumbs

1 teaspoon cayenne pepper

Sea salt to taste

Black pepper to taste

Skinny Secret

Casseroles are great for large or small crowds. The best thing is that your guests will probably eat most, if not all, of the casserole, sparing you the temptation to eat all the leftovers.

1. Fill a large-quart boiler halfway with water. Add 1 teaspoon salt. Bring to a boil and add the asparagus. Cook for 30 seconds, then drain. Set aside.

2. Preheat oven to 375°F. Spray a large round 2-quart casserole dish with nonstick cooking spray. In a bowl, whisk together the eggs, egg whites, and milk. Add the sour cream, cheese, bread crumbs, and cayenne. Mix well. Add asparagus and season with salt and pepper to taste. Pour into prepared casserole dish.

3. Bake for 45 to 50 minutes, until the top is light brown.

SERVES 8	
Serving size	½ cup

CALORIES PER SERVING	
Original recipe	384
SYS recipe	75

NUTRITIONAL BREAKDOWN	
Fat	2g
Carbohydrates	10g
Protein	6g
Sodium	120mg

cheesy squeezy potatoes

CALORIE SAVINGS

450

When you've gotta have your cheese fix, go for this lean version by substituting nonfat milk, nonfat ricotta cheese, and nonfat cottage cheese for whole milk, whole-milk ricotta, and high-fat, high-calorie crème fraîche.

1 tablespoon olive oil

1 large shallot, peeled and diced

2 tablespoons plain flour

1¾ cups nonfat milk

1 teaspoon sea salt

1 teaspoon ground black pepper

½ cup nonfat ricotta cheese

½ cup nonfat cottage cheese

½ teaspoon dry mustard

Small pinch ground nutmeg

4 large baking potatoes, peeled and cut into ¼-inch slices

1. Preheat oven to 350°F. Prepare a small rectangular baking dish by spraying with nonstick spray. Place potatoes into large mixing bowl and set aside.

2. In a heavy saucepan, heat the oil over medium heat for a few seconds. Add the shallots and sauté until tender, about 3 minutes. Add the flour and stir to combine. Add the milk, salt, and pepper and cook until just bubbling. Add the ricotta and cottage cheese, mustard, and nutmeg, and stir to mix well. Pour the milk/cheese mixture over the potatoes and toss to coat.

3. Transfer to the prepared baking dish, cover with aluminum foil, and bake for 30 to 40 minutes. Uncover and bake for an additional 10 to 15 minutes or until the potatoes are tender.

Skinny Secret

This recipe proves that cheese and potatoes don't have to be super-fattening. Enjoy with lean Terriyummy Beef (recipe, page 83).

SERVES 10		CALORIES PER SERVING		NUTRITIONAL BREAKDOWN	
Serving size	½ cup	Original recipe	558	Fat	2g
		SYS recipe	108	Carbohydrates	18g
				Protein	5g
				Sodium	79mg

primavera risotto

A simple way to reduce calories and fat is to cut back on high-fat ingredients such as olive oil and Parmesan cheese. Focus on fresh, vibrant vegetables that are steamed or lightly sautéed, and use fat-free chicken broth, which is still packed with chicken flavor.

1 tablespoon olive oil
2 garlic cloves, chopped
½ white or yellow onion, chopped
Fine zest of 1 lemon
½ cup dry white wine such as sauvignon blanc
½ cup fresh green beans, cut into 1-inch pieces
2 Roma tomatoes, seeded and diced
½ cup frozen green peas
½ cup fresh yellow corn, cut off the cob
5 cups low-sodium, fat-free chicken broth, brought to a boil and simmering
1½ cups arborio rice
¼ cup grated Parmesan cheese
Sea salt to taste
Black pepper to taste

1. In large-quart boiler, heat the oil over medium heat. Add the garlic, onion, and lemon. Sauté until the onion is tender, about 4 minutes. Add the lemon zest, white wine, beans, tomatoes, peas, and corn. Sauté for about 2 minutes.

2. Add the rice and stir to brown, about 2 minutes. Add ½ cup of the chicken broth to rice mixture, and cook until all the moisture has been absorbed, stirring constantly. Continue adding the broth in ½-up increments until all the broth has been added. Once all broth has been added, cook until the rice is soft but still slightly al dente.

3. Stir in the cheese and season with salt and pepper. Serve in ½-cup portions.

Skinny Secret

Another cheese that tastes great in risotto is Gruyère. If you choose to substitute Gruyère for the Parmesan, use the same amount and cut it into small cubes before adding. Stir until the cheese melts and then serve. Gruyère adds only 3.5 calories and .3 grams of fat per serving!

SERVES 8	
Serving size	½ cup

CALORIES PER SERVING	
Original recipe	580
SYS recipe	107

NUTRITIONAL BREAKDOWN	
Fat	6g
Carbohydrates	6g
Protein	7g
Sodium	35mg

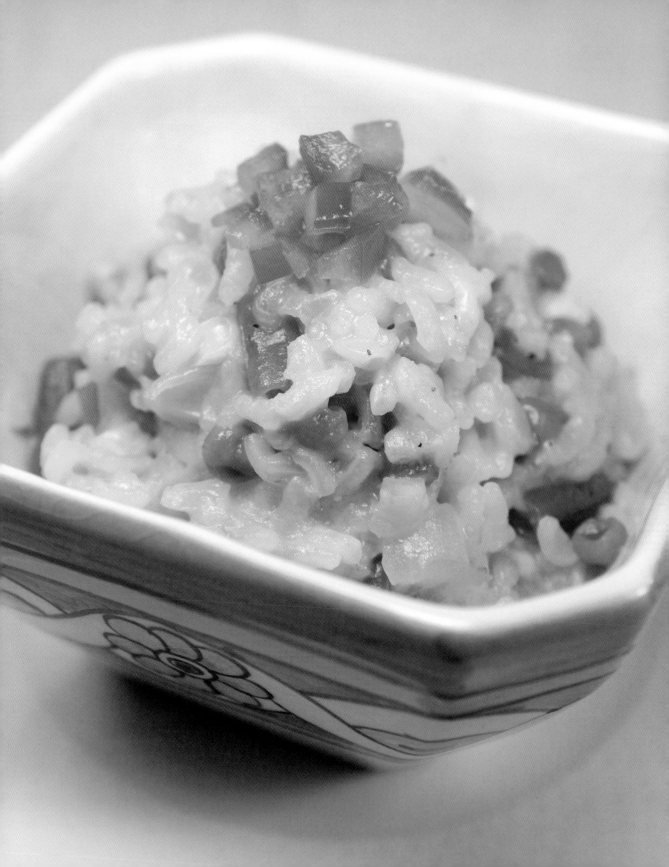

sugar-me-sweet baked beans

This Southern-style recipe tastes even more delicious with the calories you save by substituting sugar-free maple syrup and lean turkey bacon for the full-fat versions.

Nonstick cooking spray
1 white onion, diced
2 (16-ounce) cans original-style baked beans
3 tablespoons prepared yellow mustard
¼ cup sugar-free maple syrup
2 tablespoons brown sugar
1 tablespoon applesauce
¼ cup ketchup
Juice of 1 lemon
4 slices turkey bacon

Skinny Secret

Using applesauce is a great way to incorporate sweet flavor into your dish. It also adds texture and helps keep foods moist.

1. Preheat oven to 350°F. Spray a large-quart casserole dish with nonstick spray. Add the onion, beans, mustard, syrup, sugar, applesauce, ketchup, and lemon. Mix well. Top with the sliced bacon.

2. Bake, uncovered, for about 45 minutes to 1 hour. Serve in ½-cup portions.

SERVES 8		CALORIES PER SERVING		NUTRITIONAL BREAKDOWN	
Serving size	½ cup	Original recipe	461	Fat	2g
		SYS recipe	165	Carbohydrates	33g
				Protein	8g
				Sodium	722mg

cajun red beans and rice

CALORIE SAVINGS
218

Most of the fat in traditional red beans and rice is in the sausage. Using low-fat turkey sausage saves over 6 grams of fat per serving!

Nonstick cooking spray

½ white or yellow onion, chopped

2 celery stalks, chopped

1 green bell pepper, seeded and chopped

2 cloves garlic, chopped

¼ pound low-fat ground turkey sausage

2 (15-ounce) cans dark red kidney beans, drained and rinsed

1 (8-ounce) can tomato sauce

1 tablespoon tomato paste

1 teaspoon Worcestershire sauce

1 teaspoon chopped fresh thyme leaves

1 teaspoon chopped fresh Italian flat-leaf parsley leaves

1 teaspoon sherry wine

4 cups hot cooked white rice

Hot pepper sauce to taste (optional)

Skinny Secret

Green leafy herbs have essential vitamins and minerals, including vitamins A, C, and K, similar to green leafy vegetables, such as spinach.

1. Spray a large skillet or saucepan with nonstick spray. Heat on medium, and add the onion and celery; sauté until tender, about 4 minutes. Add the bell pepper and garlic, and sauté for an additional 3 to 4 minutes. Add the sausage and cook until browned, about 4 minutes. Add the beans, tomato sauce, tomato paste, and Worcestershire. Stir to combine. Then, stir in the thyme, parsley, and sherry.

2. Reduce heat, cover, and simmer for about 25 minutes, adding ¼ cup water if needed. Spoon ¼- to ½-cup servings over ½ cup cooked rice.

SERVES 8	
Serving size	½ cup

CALORIES PER SERVING	
Original recipe	383
SYS recipe	165

NUTRITIONAL BREAKDOWN	
Fat	1g
Carbohydrates	29g
Protein	11g
Sodium	284mg

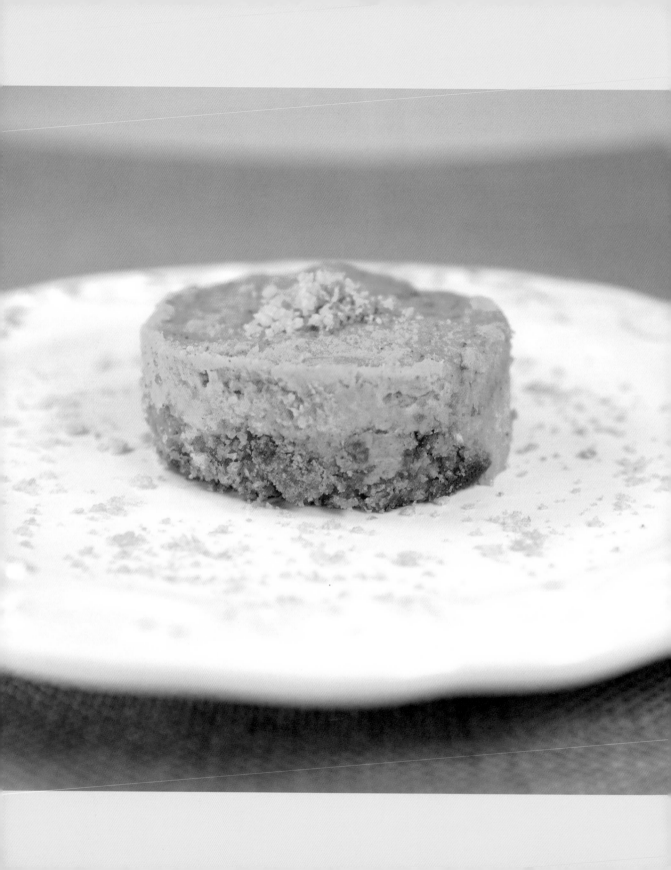

sweet-as-pie sweet potatoes

Southern-style sweet potato casserole traditionally has marshmallows with a sugary, buttery crust on the top. Here, the crust is lighter and on the bottom, like a soufflé, and the marshmallows aren't needed at all for these naturally sweet, sweet potatoes.

Nonstick cooking spray

1 cup unsweetened cornflakes, crushed

1 tablespoon brown sugar

4 large sweet potatoes, peeled and cut into 2-inch cubes

2 tablespoons butter, softened

¼ cup granulated sugar

2 tablespoons honey

1 teaspoon ground cinnamon

¼ teaspoon ground nutmeg

1 (5-ounce) can fat-free evaporated milk

1 teaspoon vanilla extract

1 egg, beaten

3 egg whites, beaten

Skinny Secret

Although canned sweet potatoes are readily available and convenient, for maximum nutrition, fresh is best.

1. Preheat oven to 350°F. Prepare a deep quart casserole dish by spraying with nonstick spray. In small mixing bowl, combine the cornflakes and sugar. Press into the bottom of the prepared baking dish.

2. Add the sweet potatoes to a large-quart boiler and fill with enough water to cover. Boil the potatoes until tender, about 20 minutes. Drain well. Return the potatoes to the boiler and mix with the butter, sugar, honey, cinnamon, nutmeg, milk, vanilla, egg, and egg whites. Mix well.

3. Pour into the prepared baking dish. Bake for 45 minutes to 1 hour. Serve in ½-cup portions.

SERVES 8	
Serving size	½ cup

CALORIES PER SERVING	
Original recipe	356
SYS recipe	148

NUTRITIONAL BREAKDOWN	
Fat	4g
Carbohydrates	25g
Protein	4g
Sodium	122mg

sweetly sweet corn bread

Cornbread recipes are often high in sugar and use whole milk or buttermilk. Using honey and nonfat milk in this recipe cuts down on both fat and calories. However, still enjoy it in moderation because cornmeal, as is most flour, is high in carbs.

Nonstick cooking spray

¾ cup yellow cornmeal

1 teaspoon honey

1 teaspoon sea salt

1 pinch black pepper

2½ cups nonfat milk

¼ teaspoon cayenne pepper

2 egg yolks

1 tablespoon butter

½ teaspoon baking powder

3 egg whites

Skinny Secret

Another delicious substitute for full-fat buttermilk is richly flavored nonfat or reduced-fat buttermilk. Believe it or not, that adds only 2 calories more per serving than the nonfat milk!

1. Preheat oven to 350°F. Spray a 9" × 13" baking dish with nonstick spray. In a medium-quart boiler over medium heat, combine the cornmeal, honey, salt, and pepper. Stir in the milk and cayenne, and heat until the mixture is thickened, about 15 minutes, stirring continually. In small bowl, whisk the egg yolks and stir quickly into the cornmeal mixture. Stir in the butter until it is melted. Turn off heat.

2. In a mixing bowl, beat together the baking powder and egg whites until stiff peaks form. Gently fold the egg whites into the cornmeal mixture. Spoon the cornmeal mixture into the prepared baking dish and bake for 40 minutes or until lightly browned and puffy. Serve hot.

SERVES 8		CALORIES PER SERVING		NUTRITIONAL BREAKDOWN	
Serving size	1 "square," about ½ cup	Original recipe	179	Fat	3g
		SYS recipe	108	Carbohydrates	12g
				Protein	5g
				Sodium	402mg

refreshingly delicious pasta salad

Many pasta salads use creamy Italian dressings, which have on average 12 grams of fat per serving. Making your own light vinaigrette gives you just over 2 fat grams per serving. As well, most pasta salads are heavy on Parmesan or other cheeses. Skip the cheese altogether to save a maximum amount of calories. If you must have cheese, substitute a nonfat shredded mozzarella cheese in small portions; about 1 tablespoon per serving is all you need for a little extra flavor.

8 ounces dried rotini pasta

¼ cup chopped red onion

1 cup chopped broccoli florets

½ cup chopped red bell pepper

½ cup chopped yellow bell pepper

1 cup chopped yellow squash

¼ cup sliced black olives

1 tablespoon extra-virgin olive oil

2 tablespoons apple cider vinegar

Sea salt to taste

Black pepper to taste

1. Prepare the pasta as directed on the package. Transfer to large mixing bowl and toss with the onion, broccoli, bell peppers, squash, and black olives.

2. In a small bowl, whisk together the oil and vinegar. Pour over the pasta and toss. Season with salt and pepper, and toss to combine. Serve in ½-cup portions.

Skinny Secret

Try using balsamic, white wine, red wine, or champagne vinegars, each of which has little or no fat or calories, to make other vinaigrettes.

SERVES 8	
Serving size	½ cup

CALORIES PER SERVING	
Original recipe	170
SYS recipe	136

NUTRITIONAL BREAKDOWN	
Fat	4g
Carbohydrates	23g
Protein	4g
Sodium	28mg

penne "lasagna" with beef

Replacing lasagna noodles with whole-wheat penne pasta versus regular penne saves on average 100 calories per recipe!

8 ounces dried whole-wheat penne pasta

1 tablespoon olive oil

¼ pound lean ground beef

¼ white onion, chopped

¼ green bell pepper, chopped

1 (15-ounce) can tomato sauce

1 (8-ounce) can stewed tomatoes

2 tablespoons tomato paste

½ cup nonfat ricotta cheese

½ cup reduced-fat mozzarella cheese

1 tablespoon grated Parmesan cheese

¼ teaspoon garlic powder

¼ teaspoon dried oregano

Sea salt to taste

Black pepper to taste

Skinny Secret

Penne pasta is delicious with just about everything. Make this dish even leaner with lean ground turkey or enjoy simply vegetarian style and leave out the beef altogether.

1. Cook pasta as directed on package, reserving ½ cup of pasta water. Drain; drizzle with the olive oil and set aside. In a large saucepan over medium heat, sauté the ground beef and onion until the beef is browned and the onion is tender, about 6 minutes. Add the bell pepper, tomato sauce, tomatoes, paste, ricotta, mozzarella, and Parmesan, and stir well to combine. Stir in the garlic powder and oregano. Add salt and pepper to taste.

2. Reduce heat to low, cover, and simmer for about 25 minutes so flavors can blend. Add reserved pasta water in ¼-cup increments if needed. When ready to serve, toss the tomato sauce with the pasta. Serve in ½-cup portions.

SERVES 8		CALORIES PER SERVING		NUTRITIONAL BREAKDOWN	
Serving size	½ cup	Original recipe	550	Fat	3g
		SYS recipe	90	Carbohydrates	46g
				Protein	7g
				Sodium	441mg

lite me up potato salad

CALORIE SAVINGS

242

Substituting nonfat yogurt for heavy, fat-laden mayonnaise saves on both fat and calories. Plus, the yogurt adds a creamier flavor than nonfat mayonnaise.

1 teaspoon chopped fresh mint leaves
¼ cup nonfat plain yogurt
1 teaspoon fresh lemon juice
1 teaspoon honey
¼ teaspoon ground mustard
2 pounds unpeeled red potatoes, cubed and boiled until just tender
½ cup chopped celery
¼ cup chopped dill pickles
¼ cup chopped red bell peppers
¼ cup chopped yellow bell peppers
¼ white onion, chopped
Sea salt to taste
Black pepper to taste

1. In a small mixing bowl, whisk together the mint, yogurt, lemon, honey, and mustard. In a large mixing bowl, combine the potatoes, celery, dill pickles, bell peppers, and onion.

2. Spoon the yogurt mixture over the potato mixture and toss to combine. Season with salt and pepper to taste. Serve in ½-cup portions.

Skinny Secret

Fresh herbs such as cilantro or Italian flat-leaf parsley are equally delicious and can be substituted for the fresh mint leaves.

SERVES 10	
Serving size	½ cup

CALORIES PER SERVING	
Original recipe	305
SYS recipe	63

NUTRITIONAL BREAKDOWN	
Fat	0
Carbohydrates	14g
Protein	2g
Sodium	74mg

nutty rice pilaf

Brown rice is healthier for you overall than white rice because it is lower in calories, higher in fiber, and slightly higher in protein. And we use almonds, which are one of the leanest nuts, with 164 calories and 14 grams of fat per 2-ounce serving.

½ tablespoon olive oil
¼ cup almonds, left whole
1 clove garlic, minced
2 green onions, chopped
Fine zest of ½ lemon
1 teaspoon chopped fresh cilantro leaves
1 cup long-grain brown rice
2¼ cups water
Sea salt to taste
Black pepper to taste

1. In a medium saucepan, heat the oil over medium heat. Add the nuts and garlic and sauté for about 1 minute. Add the onion, lemon zest, and cilantro. Stir to combine. Add the rice, stir well, and cook for about 1 minute. Add the water, stir, and bring to a boil.

2. Cover and reduce heat. Let simmer until the rice is cooked, about 40 minutes. When the rice is done, season with salt and pepper to taste. Serve in ½-cup portions.

Skinny Secret

Nuts in general are good for you in moderation. Cashews, walnuts, and hazelnuts are all good alternatives to almonds in this recipe.

SERVES 4		CALORIES PER SERVING		NUTRITIONAL BREAKDOWN	
Serving size	½ cup	Original recipe	333	Fat	3g
		SYS recipe	189	Carbohydrates	36g
				Protein	4g
				Sodium	3mg

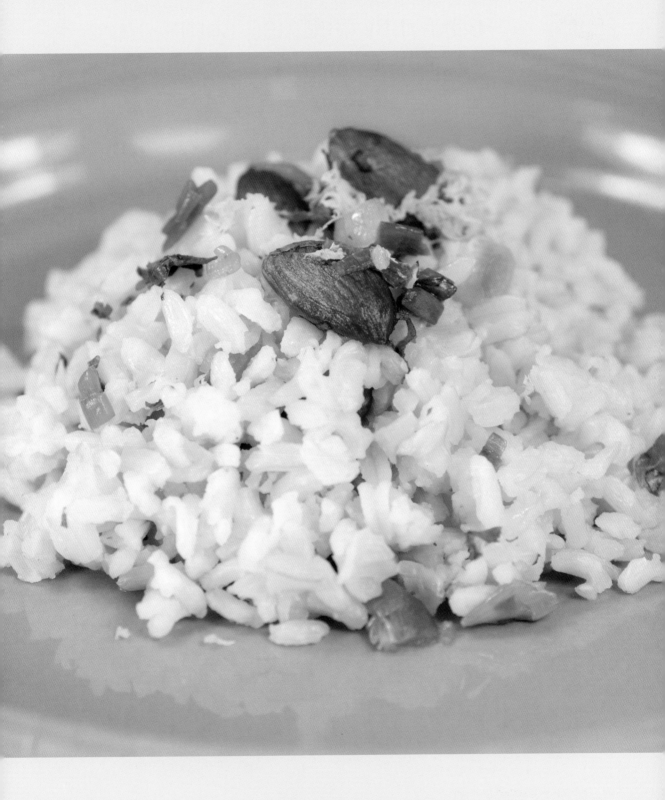

orzo with creamed corn

Cutting back on the oil and using reduced-fat cheese keep this recipe slimming for your figure.

8 ounces orzo pasta

3 large cucumbers, peeled, seeded, and diced

1½ cups reduced-fat feta cheese

2 tablespoons extra-virgin olive oil

½ tablespoon red wine vinegar

2 cups fresh yellow corn

¼ red onion, chopped

1 tablespoon chopped fresh cilantro leaves

1 tablespoon chopped kalamata olives

Sea salt to taste

Black pepper to taste

1. Prepare the orzo as directed on the package until al dente. Drain.

2. In a food processor, combine ½ of the cucumbers, 1 cup of the cheese, the oil, vinegar, and 1 cup of the corn. Process until smooth.

3. Toss the orzo with the remaining cucumber, cheese, corn, onion, cilantro, and olives. Add the dressing and toss to coat. Season to taste with salt and pepper. Serve immediately or chill for 1 hour and serve.

Skinny Secret

This makes a great entrée salad as well as a side dish. If you like, add freshly chopped broccoli florets and diced red bell pepper for more flavor and color without adding fat or calories.

SERVES 8	
Serving size	¾ cup

CALORIES PER SERVING	
Original recipe	272
SYS recipe	212

NUTRITIONAL BREAKDOWN	
Fat	7g
Carbohydrates	30g
Protein	9g
Sodium	312mg

gratis gratin with broccoli and cheese

Keep fat away with this low-calorie version by substituting nonfat sour cream, nonfat cream cheese, reduced-fat Swiss cheese, and using nonstick cooking spray as opposed to butter.

Nonstick cooking spray

1 teaspoon salt

5 cups broccoli florets, large ones cut in half, smaller pieces left whole

½ tablespoon olive oil

1 white or yellow onion, chopped

½ cup sliced cremini mushrooms

Fine zest of ½ lemon

Juice of ½ lemon

Sea salt and black pepper to taste

¼ cup nonfat sour cream

½ cup nonfat cream cheese, softened

½ cup reduced-fat shredded Swiss cheese

2 tablespoons grated Parmesan cheese

Skinny Secret

This recipe can be made with fresh cauliflower, green beans, or zucchini.

1. Preheat oven to 400°F. Spray a 9" × 13" baking dish with nonstick spray. Fill a large-quart boiler halfway with water. Add 1 teaspoon salt. Bring to a boil. Add the broccoli and let cook for 30 seconds. Strain well and discard the liquid.

2. In a large saucepan, heat the olive oil over medium heat. Add the onion and mushrooms, lemon zest and juice, and season lightly with salt and pepper; sauté for about 5 minutes. Remove from heat.

3. In a mixing bowl, combine the sour cream, cream cheese, and Swiss cheese. Add the broccoli and onion mixture. Toss well to coat. Pour into the prepared baking dish and sprinkle with the Parmesan cheese. Bake for about 25 minutes or until the top is lightly browned.

SERVES 10		CALORIES PER SERVING		NUTRITIONAL BREAKDOWN	
Serving size	½ cup	Original recipe	104	Fat	1g
		SYS recipe	52	Carbohydrates	6g
				Protein	5g
				Sodium	151mg

spinning-spinach stuffed mushrooms

Lower-fat, lower-calorie turkey bacon and nonfat milk and sour cream are all great ways to knock out calories without sacrificing flavor.

2 slices turkey bacon
½ white or yellow onion, chopped
1 clove garlic, minced
Squeeze of lemon juice
1 teaspoon chopped fresh thyme leaves
1 (10-ounce) package frozen spinach, thawed and drained
½ cup nonfat milk
½ cup nonfat sour cream
Sea salt to taste
Black pepper to taste
12 large button mushrooms, stems removed
2 tablespoons grated Parmesan cheese

Skinny Secret

These make great appetizers for parties. Use the smaller cremini mushrooms for appetizers. You can also substitute baby portobellos or large portobellos for an entrée-sized serving!

1. Preheat oven to 400°F. Line a baking sheet with parchment paper or spray with nonstick cooking spray. In a skillet over medium heat, cook the bacon until crisp. Remove and drain on paper towels. Wipe the grease out of the skillet, leaving some for the rest of the recipe.

2. Return the skillet to the heat and add the onion, garlic, lemon, and thyme. Sauté until the flavors combine and the onion is tender, about 6 minutes. Add the spinach and sauté for about 5 minutes. Stir in the milk and sour cream until blended and smooth. Season with salt and pepper. Chop or crumble the bacon into small pieces.

3. Stuff each mushroom with ½ to 1 tablespoon of the spinach mixture. Top with bacon crumbles and a pinch of Parmesan cheese.

4. Bake for about 12 minutes, or until the top is browned slightly and the mushrooms are just tender.

SERVES 12	
Serving size	1 mushroom

CALORIES PER SERVING	
Original recipe	174
SYS recipe	30

NUTRITIONAL BREAKDOWN	
Fat	.3g
Carbohydrates	4g
Protein	3g
Sodium	126mg

potato lat-kiss

Most of the fat in latkes comes from the oil. Lightly frying and then baking helps to keep them lean.

1½ pounds large russet baking potatoes, peeled
1 large shallot, minced
¼ cup whole-wheat flour
2 egg whites
1 pinch white pepper
3 tablespoons light canola oil

1. Preheat oven to 450°F. Line a baking sheet with parchment paper or spray with nonstick spray. Shred the potatoes and shallot in a food processor or using a mandoline. Transfer to a colander to drain, squeezing the mixture to extract as much liquid as possible. Transfer to a large mixing bowl and gently add the flour, egg whites, and pepper, tossing until just combined. Form into 2½-inch flattened rounds.

2. Heat the oil in a heavy skillet over medium-high heat. Add the latkes and brown on each side, about 1 minute per side. Drain on paper towels, then transfer to the prepared baking sheet. Bake until crisp, about 7 to 8 minutes. Serve hot.

Skinny Secret

Whole-wheat flour and egg whites are best for reducing calories, fat, and cholesterol and increasing fiber.

SERVES 10	
Serving size	1 latke

CALORIES PER SERVING	
Original recipe	192
SYS recipe	100

NUTRITIONAL BREAKDOWN	
Fat	4g
Carbohydrates	14g
Protein	3g
Sodium	15mg

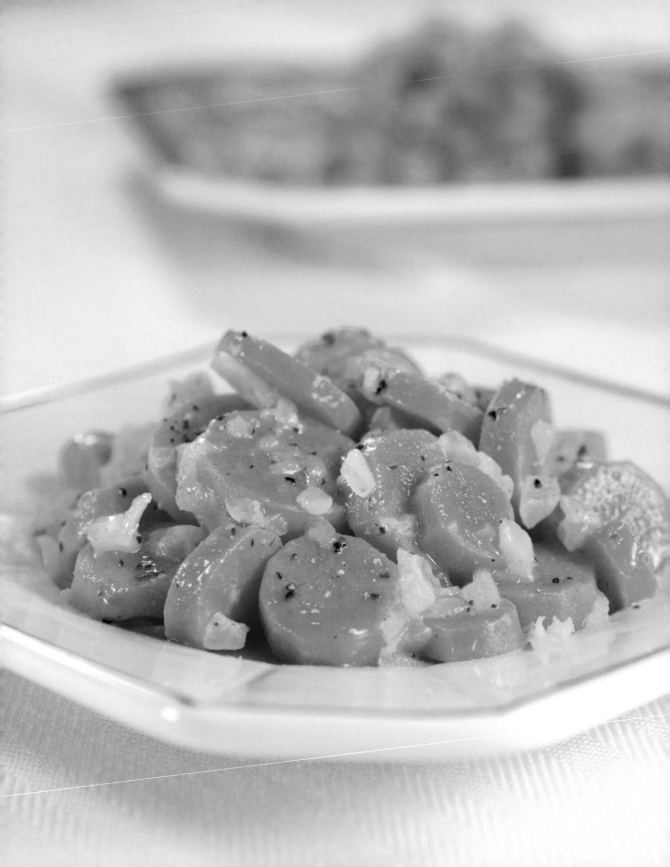

glazed carrots

Glazed carrots are usually topped with heavy doses of sugar. Substitute sugar-free maple syrup and also reduce the amount of butter and syrup you use. In this delicious recipe, a little goes a long way and the flavor is maximized by the spiciness of the Dijon mustard.

3 cups sliced carrots
1 tablespoon butter
¾ white onion, chopped
2 tablespoons sugar-free maple syrup
1 teaspoon prepared Dijon mustard
Sea salt to taste
Black pepper to taste

1. Fill a medium-quart boiler halfway with water. Add the carrots and bring to a boil. Cook until just tender, but still slightly firm. Do not overcook or the carrots with become mushy. Drain and set aside.

2. In a large saucepan over medium heat, melt the butter. Add the onion and sauté until slightly tender, about 3 minutes. Stir in the syrup and mustard. Combine well and then add the carrots, stirring to coat. Serve warm.

Skinny Secret

If you don't have sugar-free maple syrup, you can make your own low-sugar "syrup" by using 1 tablespoon of brown sugar mixed with 1 tablespoon of applesauce.

SERVES 4		CALORIES PER SERVING		NUTRITIONAL BREAKDOWN	
Serving size	½ cup	Original recipe	130	Fat	3g
		SYS recipe	84	Carbohydrates	15g
				Protein	1g
				Sodium	125mg

fry-me-not fried rice

Using peanut oil adds flavor, and peanut oil has slightly less fat than canola or vegetable oil. Using only the egg whites saves on nearly 4 grams of fat per serving.

1½ tablespoons peanut oil

1 tomato, seeded and diced

2 teaspoons low-sodium soy sauce

1 clove garlic, minced

3 green onions, chopped

4 cremini mushrooms, sliced

1 teaspoon fish sauce

1½ teaspoons red pepper flakes

1 cup cooked white rice

Juice of 1 lime

¼ cup cooked bay shrimp

2 egg whites

Skinny Secret

You can vary this recipe by adding shredded carrots, beef, pork, or chicken.

1. In a wok or large saucepan, heat the oil over medium-high heat. Add the tomato, soy sauce, garlic, onions, and mushrooms. Sauté for about 2 minutes. Add the fish sauce, pepper flakes, and rice. Stir until combined, and cook for about 2 minutes. Add the lime and shrimp, and stir. Add the egg whites and cook, stirring quickly, about 2 minutes.

2. Serve in ½-cup portions as a side dish.

SERVES 2		CALORIES PER SERVING		NUTRITIONAL BREAKDOWN	
Serving size	½ cup	Original recipe	377	Fat	11g
		SYS recipe	266	Carbohydrates	28g
				Protein	14g
				Sodium	931mg

i'm not dreamin' polenta cake

This recipe can be made so many ways, but is most often made with lots of butter and heavy cream. Here, the butter is skipped altogether and nonfat milk is used along with some reduced-fat cheese.

Nonstick cooking spray

3¼ cups water

1½ cups yellow cornmeal or polenta

¼ cup nonfat milk

1 teaspoon chopped fresh thyme leaves

1 teaspoon chopped fresh rosemary leaves

1 pinch sea salt

1 pinch black pepper

½ cup shredded reduced-fat mozzarella cheese

1. Preheat oven to 375°F. Spray a 9-inch square baking dish with nonstick spray. In a large-quart boiler, bring the water to a boil over medium-high heat. Gradually stir in the cornmeal. Stirring constantly, bring to a boil and stir until thickened. Stir in the milk, thyme, and rosemary. Season lightly with salt and pepper. Stir until thickened. When thick, stir in the cheese until melted.

2. Pour the mixture into the prepared baking dish and bake for 30 minutes or until the top is lightly golden. Cut into 8 squares and serve.

Skinny Secret

This dish can also be used as an appetizer. Cut into 16 squares and top with a slice of seared fresh tuna, grilled chicken, or blackened salmon.

SERVES 8	
Serving size	1 (2-inch) square, about ½ cup

CALORIES PER SERVING	
Original recipe	533
SYS recipe	133

NUTRITIONAL BREAKDOWN	
Fat	3g
Carbohydrates	21g
Protein	7g
Sodium	55mg

everything's bloomin' with delicious onions and bacon

This style of onion is usually thickly battered and deep-fried, making it full of unwanted fat and calories. This baked version is light and delicious and makes a great conversation piece for dinner parties. Squeeze a little lemon juice on it when serving, if desired.

2 large Vidalia or other sweet onions
¼ cup plain bread crumbs
½ teaspoon sea salt
½ teaspoon black pepper
¼ teaspoon cayenne pepper
¼ teaspoon ground mustard
1 slice turkey bacon, cooked crisp and crumbled

Skinny Secret

Avoid eating deep-fried foods whenever possible. They are filled with saturated fat, loaded with calories, and are just not worth the temporary satisfaction. Baked versions like this one are equally, if not more, delicious, and you can enjoy them guilt-free!

1. Preheat oven to 400°F. Line a baking sheet with parchment paper or spray with nonstick spray. Slice the onions into "petals": Trim the "top" slightly. Peel off the skin. Slice down from the top to the stem, stopping about 1 inch before bottom, or root, leaving the onion intact. Slice 5 times, making 10 sections. Gently pull the "petals" apart slightly.

2. Place the bread crumbs, salt, black pepper, cayenne, and mustard in a large plastic bag. Toss to mix. Spray the onions with nonstick spray. Add 1 onion to the bag and toss to coat. Remove from the bag and transfer to the prepared baking sheet. Coat the other onion and place on the baking sheet. Top each onion with ½ of the bacon crumbles.

3. Bake until tender, about 40 minutes. Serve ½ onion per person.

SERVES 4		CALORIES PER SERVING		NUTRITIONAL BREAKDOWN	
Serving size	½ onion	Original recipe	577	Fat	8g
		SYS recipe	36	Carbohydrates	6g
				Protein	15g
				Sodium	128mg

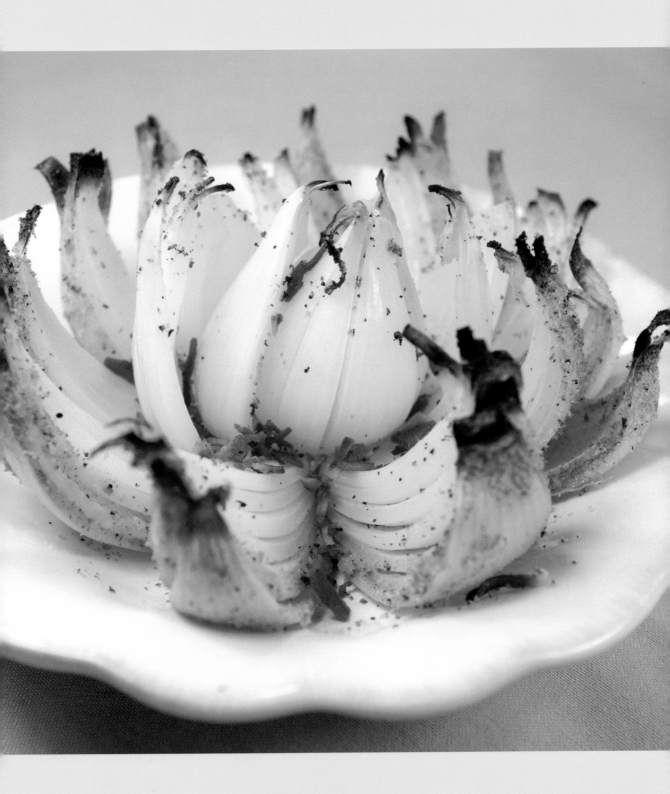

brussels with cheese

These nutritious Brussels sprouts are lean and flavorful with the substitution of lower-calorie turkey bacon and reduced-fat feta cheese.

1 pound Brussels sprouts, stems trimmed
½ cup water
Juice of 1 lemon
Sea salt to taste
2 slices turkey bacon, chopped into ½-inch pieces
½ large onion, chopped
½ tablespoon Dijon mustard
¼ cup dry white wine such as sauvignon blanc
¼ cup reduced-fat feta cheese
Black pepper to taste

Skinny Secret

Brussels sprouts are very good for you, providing over 18 mg of calcium and over 171 mg of potassium in a ½-cup serving.

1. Preheat broiler. Place the Brussels sprouts in a large-quart boiler over medium-high heat with the water, lemon, and a pinch of salt. Bring to a simmer, cover, and let simmer for about 10 minutes. Drain and cut the Brussels sprouts in half.

2. Cook the bacon in a heavy ovenproof skillet until crisp. Add the onion and sauté until tender. Add the mustard and wine, and stir until combined and all the ingredients are mixed well. Add the Brussels sprouts. Sauté for about 5 minutes. Stir in the cheese. Add pepper to taste.

3. Transfer the skillet to the broiler. Broil for about 1 minute, just until the Brussels sprouts are slightly browned. Serve in ½-cup portions.

SERVES 4		CALORIES PER SERVING		NUTRITIONAL BREAKDOWN	
Serving size	½ cup	Original recipe	297	Fat	2g
		SYS recipe	83	Carbohydrates	15g
				Protein	7g
				Sodium	322mg

guilt-free snacks and appetizers

spinach artichoke dip

This party favorite really loads up on the calories. Enjoy your party guilt-free by substituting nonfat mayonnaise and sour cream!

Nonstick cooking spray
1 (14-ounce) can artichoke hearts, drained and chopped
4 cups frozen chopped spinach, thawed and drained
1 8-ounce can water chestnuts, drained and chopped
1½ cups nonfat mayonnaise
½ cup grated Parmesan cheese
1½ cups nonfat sour cream
2 cloves fresh garlic, chopped
2 green onions, roots trimmed, green and white parts chopped
1 teaspoon cayenne pepper

Preheat oven to 375°F. Spray a 1-quart baking dish with nonstick spray. In a large mixing bowl, combine all the ingredients and mix well. Transfer to the prepared baking dish and bake, uncovered, for 45 minutes. Cover the dish with aluminum foil and bake for an additional 15 minutes.

Skinny Secret

This dip is usually served with high-calorie, high-fat tortilla chips. Although substituting nonfat mayonnaise and nonfat sour cream saves a ton of calories and fat in this recipe, save even more calories by dipping with cucumber slices or endive leaves, or use more healthy, lower-in-fat Melba rounds or saltine crackers.

SERVES 6		CALORIES PER SERVING		NUTRITIONAL BREAKDOWN	
Serving size	½ cup	Original recipe	400	Fat	1g
		SYS recipe	214	Carbohydrates	24g
				Protein	9g
				Sodium	1,270mg

lite 'n' creamy vanilla pudding pop

Keeping sugar content low and substituting nonfat milk for the usual whole milk makes all the difference in this delicious snack!

2 tablespoons granulated sugar

⅓ cup honey

¼ cup cornstarch

¼ teaspoon sea salt

3 cups nonfat milk

3 egg yolks

2 teaspoons vanilla extract

*Special equipment needed: 3-ounce pop tray and wooden sticks

1. In a double-boiler over medium heat, whisk together the sugar, honey, cornstarch, and salt. Gradually whisk in the milk, mixing until all the ingredients are dissolved and combined. Whisk in the egg yolks. Whisk constantly, cooking until the first bubbles appear (this may take 5 minutes or so). Continue to whisk for 1 minute.

2. Remove from heat and stir in the vanilla. Divide the mixture among the pop molds. Chill in the refrigerator until cool and thickened, about 1 hour. Insert the pop sticks, and freeze until solid, about 4 hours. Pops will keep for up to 2 weeks in the freezer. To release easily, run the molds quickly under warm (not hot) water.

Skinny Secret

Even when you are eating well, enjoying realistic portions, and consuming smaller meals throughout the day, you still sometimes crave a snack! Having quick access to a satisfying, fun, tasty, and healthy snack like this one is essential to help you avoid reaching for fattening snacks like potato chips, corn chips, or cookies.

MAKES 10 POPS		CALORIES PER SERVING		NUTRITIONAL BREAKDOWN	
Serving size	1 pop	Original recipe	169	Fat	1g
		SYS recipe	87	Carbohydrates	15g
				Protein	3g
				Sodium	42mg

three-cheese dip

If you hear about a recipe with three cheeses in it, you automatically think "off limits." Enjoy this tasty cheese dip by substituting reduced-fat Cheddar and Monterey jack cheeses and substituting nonfat cream cheese for half of the needed cream cheese.

¼ cup minced green onion

1 clove garlic, minced

2 tablespoons water

1 (14-ounce) can stewed tomatoes, drained and chopped

1 (4-ounce) can green chilies

1 teaspoon chili powder

1 dash hot pepper sauce

1 cup reduced-fat Cheddar cheese

1 cup reduced-fat pepper jack cheese

1 (3-ounce) package cream cheese, softened

1 (3-ounce) package nonfat cream cheese, softened

Skinny Secret

To keep this recipe truly low-calorie, serve with fresh vegetables such as broccoli, carrots, cucumbers, and red bell pepper slices.

1. In a large saucepan, combine the onion, garlic, and water. Sauté for about 3 minutes on medium heat. Add the tomatoes, chilies, chili powder, and hot pepper sauce. Cook, uncovered, over medium heat until hot.

2. Add the Cheddar cheese, pepper jack cheese, and cream cheese. Cook over low heat, stirring continually until the cheese is melted. Serve hot.

MAKES 2½ TO 3 CUPS	
Serving size	2 tablespoons

CALORIES PER SERVING	
Original recipe	108
SYS recipe	48

NUTRITIONAL BREAKDOWN	
Fat	4g
Carbohydrates	2g
Protein	5g
Sodium	206mg

queso dip

A great cheese dip for parties, keep this one slimming by using reduced-fat Cheddar cheese and a combination of lower-calorie and lower-fat soft Neufchâtel cheese with nonfat cream cheese. For added slimming alternatives, dip with fresh vegetables instead of fried tortilla chips.

¼ cup minced red bell pepper

1 (14-ounce) can stewed tomatoes, drained and chopped

1 (4-ounce) can green chilies

1 teaspoon chili powder

½ teaspoon dry mustard

1 dash hot pepper sauce

2 cups reduced-fat Cheddar cheese

1 (3-ounce) package Neufchâtel cheese, softened

1 (3-ounce) package nonfat cream cheese, softened

1. In a large saucepan, combine the red bell pepper, tomatoes, chilies, chili powder, mustard, and hot pepper sauce. Cook, uncovered, over medium heat until hot. Add the Cheddar, Neufchâtel, and cream cheese. Cook over low heat, stirring constantly, until the cheese is melted.

2. Serve hot with reduced-fat baked tortilla strips or freshly chopped vegetables.

Skinny Secret

This dip makes a great "sauce" for burritos, such as the Beef Lovers' Burrito on page 49.

MAKES 2½ TO 3 CUPS	
Serving size	2 tablespoons

CALORIES PER SERVING	
Original recipe	108
SYS recipe	45

NUTRITIONAL BREAKDOWN	
Fat	3g
Carbohydrates	2g
Protein	4g
Sodium	169mg

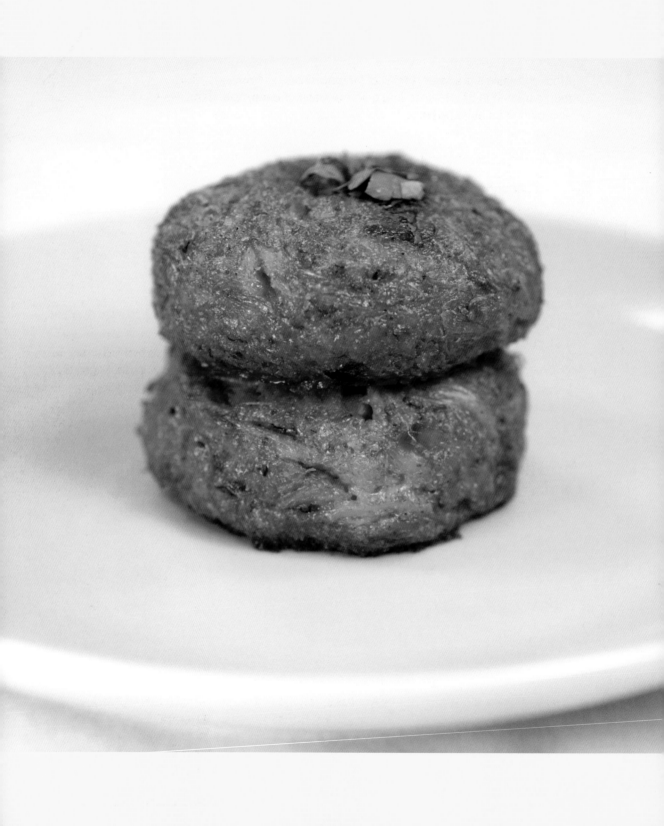

oven-baked crab cakes

Most crab cakes are made with regular mayonnaise, whole eggs, and then pan-fried in oil. These baked cakes are easy, healthy, and can also be served as appetizers.

¼ cup plus 1 tablespoon nonfat mayonnaise
½ tablespoon minced fresh cilantro leaves
½ tablespoon minced fresh Italian flat-leaf parsley leaves
½ teaspoon cayenne pepper
1 tablespoon Old Bay seasoning
2 egg whites
Fine zest of ½ lemon
¼ cup Italian-style bread crumbs
1 (1-pound) can lump crabmeat, drained

1. Preheat oven to 425°F. Line a baking sheet with parchment paper or spray with nonstick spray. In a large mixing bowl, mix together the mayonnaise, cilantro, parsley, cayenne, Old Bay seasoning, egg whites, and lemon. Mix well. Add the bread crumbs until well blended. Fold in the crabmeat until just combined.

2. Mold into 2-inch round cakes. Place on the prepared baking sheet. Bake for 12 to 15 minutes, until golden.

Skinny Secret

An easy way to flavor foods with no added fat and calories is to use citrus zest. Lemon is used here, but don't be afraid to experiment with other flavors, such as lime or orange.

SERVES 24	
Serving size	1 crab cake

CALORIES PER SERVING	
Original recipe	379
SYS recipe	22

NUTRITIONAL BREAKDOWN	
Fat	.1g
Carbohydrates	2g
Protein	4g
Sodium	178mg

wingin' it buffalo wings

Traditional buffalo wing recipes fry the chicken, which is coated with buttery, sugary sauces. In this recipe, you bake the chicken and coat it in a low-fat sauce.

1 tablespoon olive oil

2 tablespoons minced white onion

1 clove garlic, minced

2 tablespoons freshly chopped tomatoes

1 tablespoon honey

1 tablespoon butter

1 tablespoon cayenne pepper

Juice of ½ lemon

3 tablespoons hot sauce

2 tablespoons ketchup

4 chicken drummettes and 4 chicken wings

Skinny Secret

When eating chicken wings, remove the skin and dip in a low-fat sauce on the side for the optimum in calorie saving.

1. Preheat oven to 375°F. In a small-quart boiler, heat the oil on medium. Add the onion and garlic. Sauté for about 3 minutes. Add the tomatoes, honey, butter, cayenne, lemon, hot sauce, and ketchup, and stir to combine. Simmer until the sauce is thickened.

2. Line a baking sheet with parchment paper or spray with nonstick spray. Place the chicken on the baking sheet and bake for 15 minutes, or until cooked through. Remove from heat and toss with the sauce. Serve hot.

SERVES 4	
Serving size	2 wings

CALORIES PER SERVING	
Original recipe	220
SYS recipe	131

NUTRITIONAL BREAKDOWN	
Fat	10g
Carbohydrates	7g
Protein	4g
Sodium	112mg

rockin' rollin' egg rolls

CALORIE SAVINGS

108

Egg rolls are almost always deep-fried. Use the oil to add flavor to the recipe while sautéing as opposed to saturating your otherwise healthy appetizer by deep-frying.

For the filling:

⅔ cup chopped celery

⅔ cup chopped carrots

1 tablespoon fresh cilantro leaves

½ teaspoon peanut oil

⅔ cup minced green onion

½ teaspoon minced fresh ginger

1 clove minced garlic

2 cups shredded napa cabbage

1½ tablespoons low-sodium soy sauce

Juice of ¼ lemon

1 pinch black pepper

For the sauce:

¾ cup low-sodium soy sauce

6 tablespoons rice vinegar

1 tablespoon sesame oil

½ tablespoon fresh minced gingerroot

Nonstick cooking spray

14 egg roll wrappers

Skinny Secret

These can also be made in smaller portions using wonton wrappers. Serve as a party appetizer with 1 teaspoon sauce per roll.

1. Make the filling: In a food processor, combine the celery, carrots, and cilantro, and pulse to finely chop. In a large, heavy skillet, heat the peanut oil over medium heat. Add the onion, ginger, and garlic. Sauté for about 2 minutes. Add the carrot mixture and cabbage. Add the soy sauce, lemon juice, and pepper. Sauté for 1 minute. Transfer to a mixing bowl, cover, and refrigerate while you make the sauce.

continued

SERVES 14		CALORIES PER SERVING		NUTRITIONAL BREAKDOWN	
Serving size	1 roll and 1 tablespoon sauce	Original recipe	200	Fat	2g
		SYS recipe	92	Carbohydrates	18g
				Protein	4g
				Sodium	673mg

rockin' rollin' egg rolls

continued

2. Make the sauce: Whisk together the soy sauce, vinegar, sesame oil, and gingerroot.

3. Preheat oven to 425°F. Spray a baking sheet with nonstick spray. Assemble the egg rolls by placing 1 wrapper on work surface. Place 3 tablespoons of filling on the wrapper. Fold the lower corner of the wrapper over the filling. Fold in the other corners and roll up in a jellyroll fashion. Dampen the finished corner with a dab of water and lightly pinch it down to seal. Repeat with the remaining wrappers.

4. Lay the prepared egg rolls on the prepared baking sheet and bake for about 18 to 20 minutes, until golden brown. Serve the egg rolls with the sauce on the side.

wrappin' it up seafood crepes

Believe it or not, plain flour is fattening. Lighten up these crepes by substituting whole-wheat flour for half of the needed plain flour. Then use nonfat milk, nonfat sour cream, nonfat cream cheese, and reduced-fat Swiss cheese for huge calorie savings.

Nonstick cooking spray

For the crepes:

⅓ cup plain flour

⅓ cup whole-wheat flour

1 cup nonfat milk

1 tablespoon canola oil

½ teaspoon granulated sugar

¼ teaspoon baking powder

¼ teaspoon sea salt

2 egg whites

For the filling:

2 tablespoons butter

¼ cup chopped cremini mushrooms

¼ cup chopped yellow onion

1½ cups cooked bay shrimp

Juice of ½ lemon

¼ cup nonfat milk

¼ cup nonfat sour cream

6 ounces nonfat cream cheese

¾ cup reduced-fat Swiss cheese

Skinny Secret

This crepe tastes so good you can skip the Swiss cheese on the top, saving an additional 90 calories. And, for ease in preparation, make the crepes ahead and freeze them until ready to use.

1. Make the crepes: In a medium bowl, whisk together all of the crepe ingredients until smooth.

continued

SERVES 8	
Serving size	1 crepe

CALORIES PER SERVING	
Original recipe	585
SYS recipe	173

NUTRITIONAL BREAKDOWN	
Fat	6g
Carbohydrates	13g
Protein	17g
Sodium	335mg

wrappin' it up seafood crepes

continued

2. Spray a nonstick skillet with nonstick cooking spray and heat on medium. Pour ¼ cup of the batter into the skillet. Tilt the skillet to cover with batter. Cook until light brown, flip, and cook until the other side is light brown. Transfer to a plate, placing wax paper between each crepe. Cover with a towel to keep warm.

3. Make the filling: In medium-quart boiler, melt the butter over medium heat. Add the mushrooms and onions; sauté until tender, about 5 minutes. Stir in the shrimp, lemon, milk, sour cream, and cream cheese. Stir continually until the cheese is melted and all is blended.

4. Preheat broiler. Spray a 9" × 13" baking dish with nonstick spray. Assemble the crepes by spooning about ¼ cup of the shrimp mixture down the center of each crepe. Roll up. Place in the prepared baking dish. Top each with 1½ tablespoons of Swiss cheese and place under the broiler. Broil until the cheese melts. Serve hot.

beefin' it up empanadas

Empanadas are traditionally made with dough and are fried, which adds loads of fat and calories. These baked ones use low-fat wonton wrappers and fresh vegetables for a truly simple, lean, and flavorful dish.

½ pound lean ground beef

1 yellow onion, finely chopped

2 cloves garlic, finely chopped

2 teaspoons cayenne pepper

1 red bell pepper, finely chopped

¼ cup corn kernels, fresh or canned (if canned, drain)

1 tablespoon chopped fresh cilantro leaves

Sea salt to taste

Black pepper to taste

24 small wonton wrappers

1. Preheat oven to 375°F. Line a baking sheet with parchment paper or spray with nonstick spray. In a large saucepan over medium heat, combine the beef, onion, garlic, and cayenne. Cook until the beef is browned and the onion is tender, about 6 minutes. Add the bell pepper, corn, and cilantro; sauté for 5 minutes. Season with salt and pepper.

2. Assemble the empanadas by laying 1 wonton wrapper on a flat surface. Place 1 tablespoon of the beef mixture in the center of the wrapper. Spread a little water around the edges of the wrapper. Fold one side of the wrapper over the mixture and press to seal the edges together. Transfer to the prepared baking sheet. Repeat with the remaining wrappers.

3. Bake for about 15 minutes, or until golden. Serve hot.

Skinny Secret

These can be made ahead and frozen before cooking. When ready to cook, remove from the freezer and bake for about 20 minutes. They can be frozen for 2 to 3 months.

SERVES 24	
Serving size	1 empanada

CALORIES PER SERVING	
Original recipe	420
SYS recipe	44

NUTRITIONAL BREAKDOWN	
Fat	<1g
Carbohydrates	6g
Protein	4g
Sodium	53mg

vegetarian empanadas

As with the Beefin' It Up Empanadas, page 161, low-calorie, low-fat wonton wrappers are used instead of high-calorie, high-fat pastry dough to make these truly nutritious. Plus, as a bonus, they are baked instead of fried in oil.

1 tablespoon olive oil
1 yellow onion, finely chopped
2 teaspoons cayenne pepper
2 cloves garlic, finely chopped
1 red bell pepper, finely chopped
1 zucchini, diced
¼ cup corn kernels, fresh or canned (if canned, drain)
2 Roma tomatoes, seeded and diced
1 tablespoon chopped fresh cilantro leaves
Sea salt to taste
Black pepper to taste
24 small wonton wrappers

Skinny Secret

Serve this empanada along with the beef version as tasty appetizers at your party to satisfy both beef lovers and vegetarians.

1. Preheat oven to 375°F. Line a baking sheet with parchment paper or spray with nonstick spray. In a large saucepan, heat the oil over medium heat. Add the onion, cayenne, and garlic. Stir to combine, and cook until the onion is tender, about 4 minutes. Add the bell pepper, zucchini, corn, tomatoes, and cilantro. Sauté for an additional 5 minutes. Season with salt and pepper.

2. Assemble the empanadas by laying 1 wonton wrapper on a flat surface. Place 1 tablespoon of the onion mixture in the center of the wrapper. Spread a little water around the edges of the wrapper. Fold one side of the wonton over the mixture and press to seal the edges together. Transfer to the prepared baking sheet. Repeat with the remaining wrappers.

3. Bake for about 15 minutes, or until golden. Serve hot.

SERVES 24	
Serving size	1 empanada

CALORIES PER SERVING	
Original recipe	177
SYS recipe	31

NUTRITIONAL BREAKDOWN	
Fat	1g
Carbohydrates	7g
Protein	1g
Sodium	48mg

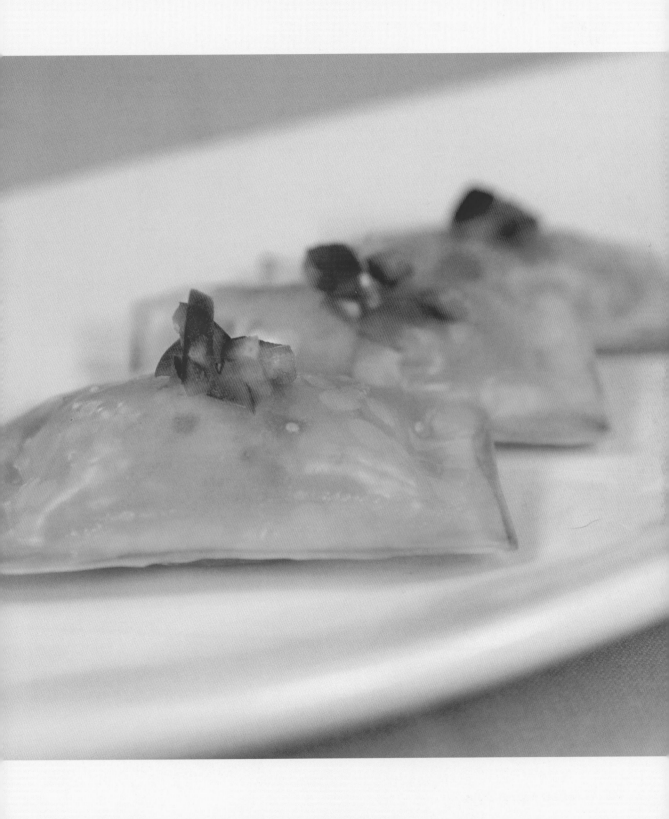

blue cheese dip

Combining high-fat foods with lower-fat or nonfat variations is a great way to keep in the flavor you love without all the calories. Here, we use nonfat cream cheese for half the needed cream cheese amount and finish with reduced-fat blue cheese crumbles. As well, leaner turkey bacon is the perfect substitution for traditional higher-fat pork bacon.

Nonstick cooking spray
6 slices lean turkey bacon
1 clove garlic, minced
1 (8-ounce) package cream cheese
2 (8-ounce) packages nonfat cream cheese
4 ounces reduced-fat blue cheese crumbles
Fine zest of ½ lemon
2 tablespoons chopped toasted walnuts

1. Preheat oven to 350°F. Spray a 1-quart round or square casserole dish with nonstick spray. In a large skillet over medium heat, cook the bacon until crisp. Drain on paper towels and crumble. Wipe out most of the oil from the skillet. Add the garlic and cook until fragrant, about 45 seconds.

2. In a large mixing bowl, cream together the cream cheese and blue cheese. Add the bacon, garlic, and lemon zest. Mix until combined. Pour the mixture into prepared casserole dish.

3. Bake for 30 to 40 minutes. Serve with freshly chopped vegetables or pita crisps.

Skinny Secret

The key to not overeating at appetizer parties is to eat a little bit before you go. Eat a healthy snack such as an apple, which is filling due to its high fiber content. One large apple provides 21 percent of your average daily recommended fiber intake.

SERVES 12		CALORIES PER SERVING		NUTRITIONAL BREAKDOWN	
Serving size	2 tablespoons	Original recipe	335	Fat	10g
		SYS recipe	149	Carbohydrates	3g
				Protein	12g
				Sodium	551mg

goat cheese soufflé

Whole-grain cereal adds flavor, texture, and fiber to this favorite dish. Keep calories low by using nonfat milk along with mostly egg whites, rather than yolks.

Nonstick cooking spray

¼ cup whole-grain cereal (such as Kashi GOLEAN Crunch!), crushed

2 tablespoons butter, softened

3½ tablespoons plain flour

2⅓ cup nonfat milk

5 ounces goat cheese

1 teaspoon chopped fresh thyme leaves

½ teaspoon chopped fresh rosemary leaves

Fine zest of ½ lemon

2 egg yolks

Sea salt to taste

Black pepper to taste

5 egg whites

1. Preheat oven to 350°F. Spray 6 (4-ounce) ramekins with nonstick spray. Press the crushed cereal lightly but evenly on the bottom and sides of the ramekins.

2. In a medium saucepan, melt the butter over medium heat. Whisk in the flour to form a paste. Cook for about 3 minutes, until light brown in color. Gradually add the milk, stirring constantly. Bring to a boil, then remove from heat. Transfer to a medium mixing bowl. Set aside.

continued

Skinny Secret

Serving in individual ramekins helps to prevent overeating. You can make mini-quiche this way as well. Just follow the quiche recipe (for example, Ginchy Quiche, recipe page 21). Line bottom of ramekins with pie crust, and pour mixture into prepared ramekins as instructed here.

SERVES 6		CALORIES PER SERVING		NUTRITIONAL BREAKDOWN	
Serving size	½ cup	Original recipe	562	Fat	13g
		SYS recipe	223	Carbohydrates	15g
				Protein	14g
				Sodium	225mg

goat cheese soufflé

continued

3. When the flour mixture is just cooled, mix in the goat cheese, thyme, rosemary, lemon zest, and egg yolks, combining well. Season with salt and pepper. Separately, beat the egg whites with mixer until stiff peaks form. Fold half of the egg whites into the goat cheese mixture, then fold in the other half. Pour the mixture into the prepared ramekins.

4. Place the ramekins in a deep baking dish filled halfway with water. Bake for 12 to 15 minutes, or until the soufflés are lightly browned. Remove the baking dish from the oven. Transfer ramekins to a baking sheet and return the ramekins to the oven (without the water bath), and bake for an additional 5 minutes. Serve hot.

cayenne shrimp dip

This dip has so much flavor from the seasoned salt and other ingredients, you won't be able to tell the difference in the substitution of nonfat mayonnaise and nonfat sour cream.

2 (11-ounce) jars unmarinated artichoke hearts, chopped
¾ cup nonfat mayonnaise
¾ cup nonfat sour cream
6 green onions, green and white parts chopped
½ tablespoon cayenne pepper
½ tablespoon chopped Italian flat-leaf parsley leaves
¾ cup cooked bay shrimp
Jane's Krazy Mixed-Up Salt (or other salt-spice blend of your choice) to taste

1. In a large mixing bowl, combine the artichokes, mayonnaise, sour cream, onions, cayenne, and parsley. Stir to combine. Gently stir in the shrimp. Season with Jane's Krazy Salt to taste.

2. Serve with freshly sliced vegetables such as cucumber, bell peppers, or endive leaves.

Skinny Secret

This recipe is so delicious that you will be tempted to eat way more than 2 tablespoons. Be sure to serve at a party so others can help you eat it, as it does not freeze well. Jane's Krazy Mixed-Up Salt is a brand of blended salt and spices that has a very unique flavor and is best for this recipe. If you cannot find it, substitute another brand of blended salt and spice.

MAKES 3 CUPS		CALORIES PER SERVING		NUTRITIONAL BREAKDOWN	
Serving size	2 tablespoons	Original recipe	110	Fat	<1g
		SYS recipe	29	Carbohydrates	4g
				Protein	2g
				Sodium	167mg

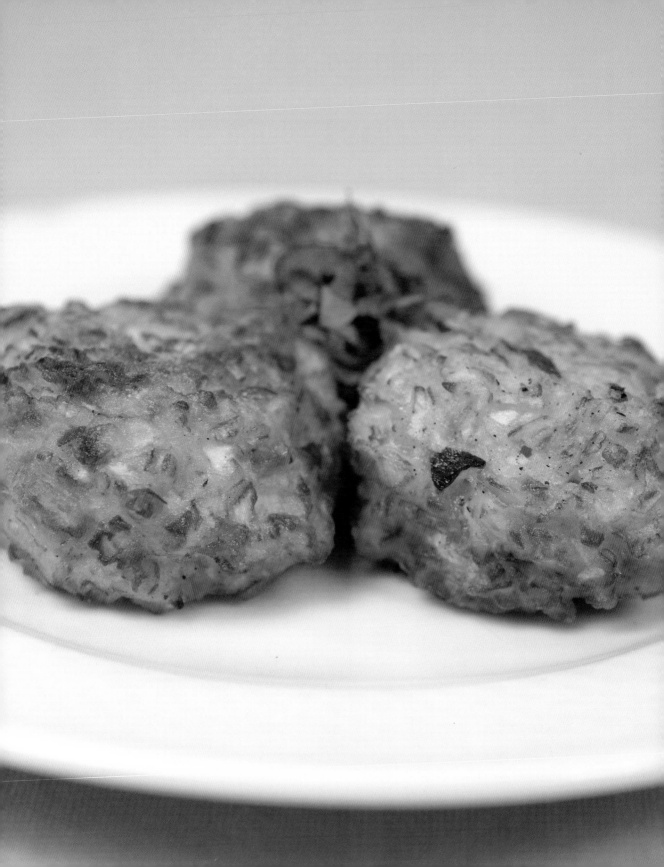

summer squash medley croquettes

Egg whites work just as well as whole eggs as a "binder" for foods—plus they save on calories, fat, and cholesterol. Even though these squash appetizers are lightly fried, they are fried in minimal amounts of oil and drained thoroughly on paper towels. As with any type of frying, make sure the oil is hot enough before adding the food product. Otherwise, your food will just soak up the unwanted oil and it won't taste good!

2 cups finely chopped yellow squash
½ cup finely chopped zucchini
1 cup finely chopped white onion
2 egg whites, lightly beaten
1 pinch sea salt
1 teaspoon cayenne pepper
1 tablespoon chopped Italian flat-leaf parsley leaves
1 pinch black pepper
¾ cup plain flour
¾ cup canola oil

Skinny Secret

If you are making this dish for a small party, cut the recipe in half so you are not tempted to overeat.

1. In a large mixing bowl, combine the yellow squash, zucchini, onion, egg whites, salt, cayenne, parsley, and black pepper, and stir to blend. Add the flour and mix until just coated. Form the mixture into 1½-inch balls.

2. Heat the oil in a heavy skillet until hot but not smoking. Add the squash balls and cook until golden and crisp, about 2 to 3 minutes. Drain on paper towels. Serve hot.

MAKES ABOUT 24 CROQUETTES	
Serving size	2 croquettes

CALORIES PER SERVING	
Original recipe	180
SYS recipe	158

NUTRITIONAL BREAKDOWN	
Fat	14g
Carbohydrates	8g
Protein	2g
Sodium	10mg

lookin' hot beef dip

Nonfat cream cheese and reduced-fat sharp Cheddar cheese are the key ingredients that make this dish lower in calories. Smoked beef is more flavorful than regular deli-style beef, so this dish is as tasty as it is slimming.

8 ounces nonfat cream cheese, softened
1¼ cups shredded reduced-fat sharp Cheddar cheese
1 tablespoon coarsely chopped fresh cilantro leaves
1 (2½-ounce) package smoked sliced beef, chopped
½ white or yellow onion, coarsely chopped
1 pinch black pepper
Sea salt (optional)

Skinny Secret

Serve this lean beef dip as a guilt-free appetizer for parties.

1. Preheat oven to 400°F. In a food processor, combine the cream cheese, Cheddar cheese, cilantro, beef, onion, and pepper. Process until smooth. Season with salt, if desired.

2. Transfer the mixture to a small baking dish. Bake until the mixture is heated through, about 10 minutes. Stir to combine, and serve.

MAKES 2 CUPS	
Serving size	2 tablespoons

CALORIES PER SERVING	
Original recipe	85
SYS recipe	51

NUTRITIONAL BREAKDOWN	
Fat	2g
Carbohydrates	1.5g
Protein	6g
Sodium	172mg

wild rice salad with raisins

Wild rice is more nutritious than white rice and is cooked here with nonfat chicken broth for added flavor without the added fat. Capitalize on the good fats and natural sugars found in almonds and golden raisins for a truly healthy dish.

1 cup long-grain white rice

1 cup wild rice

4 cups low-sodium, fat-free chicken broth

2 stalks celery, chopped

1 bunch green onions, chopped

1 cup broccoli florets, chopped

1 red bell pepper, chopped

¼ cup almonds, chopped and toasted

½ cup golden raisins

Sea salt to taste

Black pepper to taste

2 tablespoons extra-virgin olive oil

1 tablespoon balsamic vinegar

Squeeze of fresh lemon juice

Skinny Secret

Rice is a great midday pick-me-up, boasting over 17 grams of carbs per ½-cup serving. Enjoy midday when your body needs the extra energy.

1. In a large-quart boiler or rice cooker, combine the white rice, wild rice, and chicken broth. Bring to a boil. Cover, reduce heat to low, and simmer for 40 minutes or until the rice is cooked. Remove from heat and allow to cool completely. Refrigerate if necessary.

2. In a large mixing bowl, combine the cooled rice, celery, onions, broccoli, red bell peppers, almonds, and raisins. Season lightly with salt and pepper.

3. In a small bowl, whisk together the oil, vinegar, and lemon juice. Pour over the rice mixture and toss to coat. Serve in ½-cup portions.

SERVES 8	
Serving size	½ cup

CALORIES PER SERVING	
Original recipe	300
SYS recipe	252

NUTRITIONAL BREAKDOWN	
Fat	6g
Carbohydrates	44g
Protein	8g
Sodium	22mg

cute-cucumber dill dip

This simple dip is made simply slimming by substituting nonfat sour cream and nonfat cream cheese for their whole-fat counterparts.

1 large cucumber, peeled, seeded, and chopped
1 cup nonfat sour cream
1 cup nonfat cream cheese, softened
Fine zest of ½ lemon
3 tablespoons fresh dill, coarsely chopped
1 pinch sea salt

1. In a food processor, combine all the ingredients. Process until smooth. Transfer to serving bowl and chill for 1 hour before serving.

2. Serve with fresh vegetables or even as a sauce on cooked chicken breasts.

Skinny Secret

This low-fat, simple, versatile dip can also be used as a substitute for sour cream on burritos, tacos, as a sauce on chicken or pork, or even as a salad dressing. Keep in an airtight container in the refrigerator for up to 2 weeks.

MAKES 2 CUPS	
Serving size	2 tablespoons

CALORIES PER SERVING	
Original recipe	83
SYS recipe	26

NUTRITIONAL BREAKDOWN	
Fat	<1g
Carbohydrates	3g
Protein	3g
Sodium	98mg

hot 'n' spicy baked sausage cheese croquettes

Substituting the reduced-fat Bisquick product and the reduced-fat cheese is the simplest way to make this popular appetizer more slimming. Additionally, baking as opposed to cooking by the traditional frying method makes these the ultimate in skinny.

2 cups reduced-fat Bisquick baking mix
2 cups reduced-fat sharp Cheddar cheese
1 pound reduced-fat lean turkey sausage
1 teaspoon cayenne pepper

1. Preheat oven to 400°F. Line a baking sheet with parchment paper or spray with nonstick cooking spray. In a large mixing bowl, combine all the ingredients. Mix well. Form into 1-inch croquettes (balls) and place on the prepared baking sheet about 1 inch apart.

2. Bake for 20 minutes or until crisp and golden.

Skinny Secret

Make these appetizers ahead of time and freeze. When ready to bake, transfer directly from the freezer to the oven and bake for an extra 5 to 7 minutes.

MAKES 30 CROQUETTES	
Serving size	2 croquettes

CALORIES PER SERVING	
Original recipe	228
SYS recipe	146

NUTRITIONAL BREAKDOWN	
Fat	7g
Carbohydrates	12g
Protein	11g
Sodium	476mg

slidin' home bbq sliders

Lean pork is accented here by minimal sugar and maximum spice. Served on a high-fiber, whole-wheat dinner roll, this little snack is sure to please your palate and your waistline.

4-pound bone-in pork shoulder roast
Sea salt to taste
Black pepper to taste
2 tablespoons brown sugar
2 tablespoons paprika
½ tablespoon chili powder
1 teaspoon ground mustard
½ cup apple cider vinegar
1 white or yellow onion, chopped
2 cloves garlic, minced
4 sprigs fresh thyme
1 sprig fresh rosemary
4 sprigs fresh Italian flat-leaf parsley
24 small Southern-style country whole-wheat dinner rolls, split
Hot pepper sauce to taste (optional)

Skinny Secret

The acidity of the vinegar helps to break down the pork, making it super-tender for sliders—but it adds no fat or calories, only flavor.

1. Lightly season the pork with salt and pepper. In a small mixing bowl, combine the brown sugar, paprika, chili powder, and mustard; mix well. Spread the spice mixture over the pork. Pour the apple cider vinegar into a slow-cooker. Add the pork, onion, garlic, thyme, rosemary, and parsley. Cover and cook on low for 8 to 10 hours, until the pork is fork-tender. Remove the pork and shred with a fork.

2. Place about ¼ cup shredded pork onto each bun and serve.

MAKES 24 SLIDERS		CALORIES PER SERVING		NUTRITIONAL BREAKDOWN	
Serving size	1 slider	Original recipe	410	Fat	13g
		SYS recipe	244	Carbohydrates	16g
				Protein	16g
				Sodium	185mg

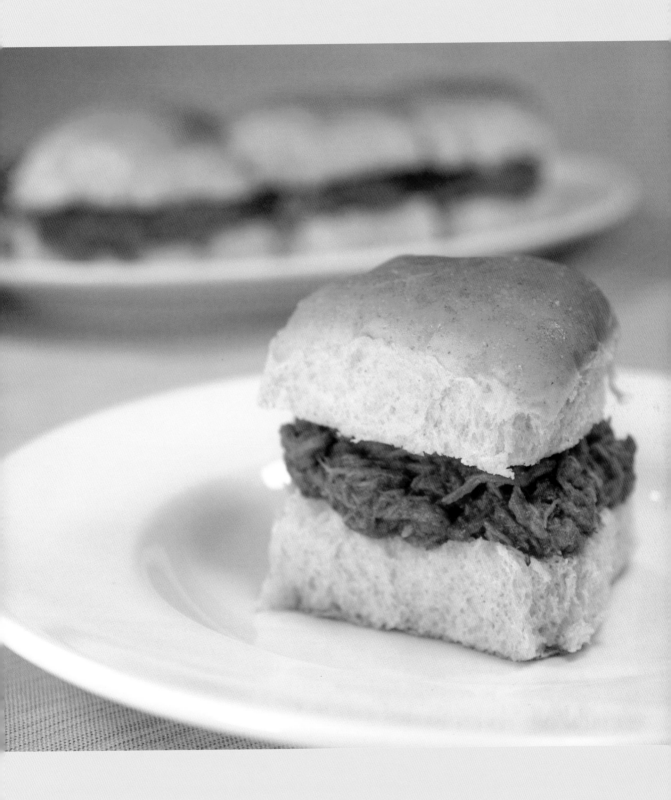

peppy pepperoncini wraps

Salami is very high in fat. Use a reduced-fat salami along with a nonfat cream cheese for an appetizer that is now very slimming. Your guests won't know the difference!

24 whole pepperoncinis
3 ounces nonfat cream cheese
Fine zest of ¼ lemon
24 slices reduced-fat salami
24 toothpicks

Using a small paring knife, slit open the sides of the pepperoncini; do not slice all the way through. In a small bowl, mix together the cream cheese and lemon zest until combined. Stuff ½ to 1 teaspoonful of cheese mixture into each pepperoncini. Wrap 1 slice of salami around the stuffed pepperoncini and secure with a toothpick.

Skinny Secret

These can be made ahead, but don't freeze them. Enjoy these light little appetizers as a snack between meals to satisfy both the sweet and spicy cravings. Just be sure to enjoy only two!

SERVES 12	
Serving size	2 "wraps"

CALORIES PER SERVING	
Original recipe	255
SYS recipe	65

NUTRITIONAL BREAKDOWN	
Fat	2g
Carbohydrates	7g
Protein	9g
Sodium	645mg

beef sliders

Combining lean ground beef with lean ground turkey saves a ton of fat and calories. When you add to that the calories and fat saved by using an egg white instead of a whole egg, and topping with reduced-fat cheese, nonfat mayonnaise, and using a mini whole-wheat bun, these sliders make entertaining fun, filling, and guilt-free.

4 ounces lean ground beef

4 ounces ground turkey

2 tablespoons yellow onion, diced

1 teaspoon Worcestershire sauce

1 clove garlic, minced

¼ teaspoon sea salt

¼ teaspoon black pepper

1 egg white

1 slice reduced-fat sharp Cheddar cheese (optional)

2 tablespoons fat-free mayonnaise

4 mini (2-inch-square) whole-wheat buns

4 slices Roma tomato

4 small lettuce leaves

Skinny Secret

Keep cooked patties on hand in the refrigerator or freezer for a super-quick lunch or snack.

1. In a mixing bowl, combine the beef, turkey, onion, Worcestershire, garlic, salt, pepper, and egg white. Mix well. Form into 4 small patties.

2. Heat a nonstick skillet on medium and add the patties. Cover, and cook for about 5 minutes. Turn the burgers, cover, and cook for an additional 5 minutes, or until cooked through. If you are adding the cheese, add ¼ slice to each patty. Cook until the cheese is melted.

3. Spread ¼ tablespoon mayonnaise on each side of the buns. Assemble the burgers using 1 slice tomato and 1 lettuce leaf for each.

SERVES 4		CALORIES PER SERVING		NUTRITIONAL BREAKDOWN	
Serving size	1 slider	Original recipe	268	Fat	6g
		SYS recipe	202	Carbohydrates	18g
				Protein	17g
				Sodium	415mg

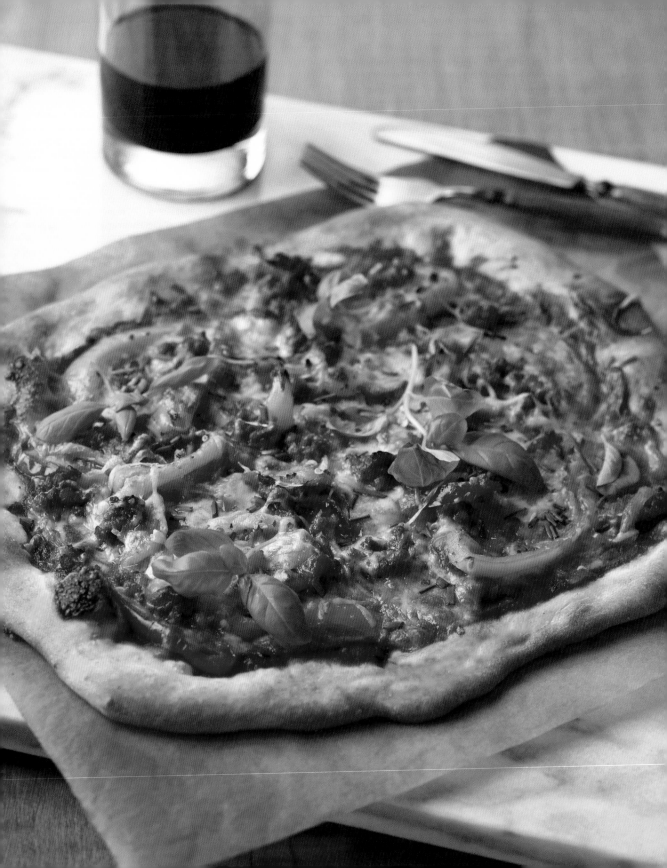

individual sausage pizza

These convenient pizza crusts are easy to use, but they do not save you a ton on fat and calories. The savings here are in the lean turkey and cheese.

¼ pound ground turkey sausage
½ white or yellow onion, chopped
½ teaspoon chopped fresh thyme leaves
1 2-crust package 8-inch Boboli pizza crusts, with sauce
½ cup reduced-fat mozzarella cheese
¼ cup chopped pitted ripe black olives

1. Preheat oven to 400°F. Line a baking sheet with parchment paper or spray with nonstick cooking spray. In a large skillet over medium heat, combine the turkey, onion, and thyme. Sauté until the turkey is browned, about 6 minutes. Drain. Spread 2 tablespoons of pizza sauce on each crust. Top each with ½ of the cooked turkey mixture. Top with cheese and black olives.

2. Place the pizzas on the prepared baking sheet and bake for 12 to 15 minutes or until the crust is crispy and the cheese is melted. Top with chopped fresh basil leaves if desired.

Skinny Secret
For an even skinnier pizza, use whole-wheat pita bread or English muffins.

SERVES 4	
Serving size	½ pizza

CALORIES PER SERVING	
Original recipe	420
SYS recipe	337

NUTRITIONAL BREAKDOWN	
Fat	12g
Carbohydrates	33g
Protein	22g
Sodium	958mg

more cheese, please mini cheese pizza

Most calories and fat in pizza are in the dough and toppings. Substitute traditional thick-crust pizza dough by using naturally high-fiber whole-wheat English muffins, and top with reduced-fat Monterey jack and Cheddar. Another cheese alternative is reduced-fat pepper jack cheese.

2 whole-wheat English muffins
4 tablespoons pizza sauce
¼ cup shredded reduced-fat Monterey jack cheese
¼ cup grated Parmesan cheese
¼ cup shredded reduced-fat Cheddar cheese

Skinny Secret

These quick, easy pizzas are just right for curbing the late afternoon hunger pains. And, they are fun for the whole family, as even kids love them.

1. Preheat oven to 375°F. Line a baking sheet with parchment paper or treat with nonstick cooking spray. Separate the English muffins into halves. Top each with 1 tablespoon of pizza sauce. In a small mixing bowl, combine the cheeses. Divide equally among each of the 4 muffin halves.

2. Bake for about 8 minutes, until the cheese is melted.

SERVES 4		CALORIES PER SERVING		NUTRITIONAL BREAKDOWN	
Serving size	1 mini pizza	Original recipe	483	Fat	5g
		SYS recipe	152	Carbohydrates	16g
				Protein	15g
				Sodium	612mg

on the bar-b bbq chicken pizza

CALORIE SAVINGS

72

Who says pizza has to be served with traditional pizza dough? Pita bread, especially whole-wheat pita if desired, is lower in calories than pizza crust. Add to your calorie savings by using skinless chicken breasts, reduced-fat BBQ sauce, and reduced-fat mozzarella cheese.

1½ cups diced cooked chicken breasts
¼ cup reduced-fat barbecue sauce
¼ cup shredded reduced-fat mozzarella cheese
4 pita pockets, left whole

1. Preheat oven to 375°F. Line a baking sheet with parchment paper or spray with nonstick cooking spray. In a small mixing bowl, toss together the chicken and barbecue sauce. Lay the pita pockets on the prepared baking sheet. Top with the chicken mixture. Top each with 1 tablespoon cheese.

2. Bake until the chicken is heated and the cheese is melted, about 5 to 7 minutes.

Skinny Secret

You can make your own BBQ sauce, but why bother when you can get tasty low-fat versions at your local store? Just be sure to find a reduced-fat variety.

SERVES 4	
Serving size	1 pita pocket pizza

CALORIES PER SERVING	
Original recipe	280
SYS recipe	208

NUTRITIONAL BREAKDOWN	
Fat	5g
Carbohydrates	18g
Protein	23g
Sodium	366mg

holy tamole guacamole

Some guacamole recipes use heavy cream or milk, but most just use fresh avocados. Although avocados taste good and are good for you, they are pretty high in fat and calories. Substituting green peas (or even green beans) for most of the avocado is a way to reduce the amount of avocado and still have a delicious-tasting guacamole.

1 teaspoon olive oil

¼ cup coarsely chopped red onion

1 clove garlic, coarsely chopped

2 tablespoons coarsely chopped fresh cilantro leaves

2 tablespoons water

1½ cups frozen peas

½ tablespoon chili powder

1 tablespoon minced jalapeño

Fine zest of 1 lemon

1 tablespoon fresh lemon juice

2 Roma tomatoes, seeded and diced

½ medium-sized ripe avocado, pitted and diced

Sea salt to taste

Black pepper to taste

Skinny Secret

If you prefer to use purely avocado and burn off the additional fat through exercise, use 6 ripe avocados for this recipe, but be aware of the extra 1,769 calories per recipe and over 162 grams of fat!

1. In a medium-quart boiler, heat the oil slightly over medium heat. Add the onion and garlic. Sauté until the onion is tender, about 3 minutes. Add the cilantro, water, and peas. Cook until the peas are tender, about 3 to 4 minutes. Purée the pea mixture in a food processor. Transfer to a mixing bowl to cool.

2. When the mixture is cool, add the chili powder, jalapeño, lemon zest, lemon juice, tomatoes, and avocado. Blend well using a fork. Season to taste with salt and pepper. Serve chilled with low-fat pita crisps or baked reduced-fat tortilla chips.

MAKES 2 CUPS	
Serving size	2 tablespoons

CALORIES PER SERVING	
Original recipe	334
SYS recipe	29

NUTRITIONAL BREAKDOWN	
Fat	1g
Carbohydrates	3g
Protein	1g
Sodium	24mg

crazy for crab salad

Crabmeat is very good for you. It's low in calories and fat, and has no carbs! Keeping it lean with veggies, spices, and nonfat ingredients is key to this slimming recipe.

4 stalks celery, diced

½ red bell pepper, diced

Fine zest of ¼ lemon

1 teaspoon lemon juice

1 tablespoon chopped fresh Italian flat-leaf parsley leaves

6 tablespoons nonfat mayonnaise

2 tablespoons nonfat sour cream

1 teaspoon Jane's Krazy Mixed-Up Salt, or sea salt to taste

½ teaspoon cayenne pepper

2 pounds lump crabmeat

1. In a medium mixing bowl, combine the celery, bell pepper, lemon zest, lemon juice, parsley, mayonnaise, sour cream, Krazy Jane, and cayenne pepper. Mix well. Stir in the crabmeat to combine.

2. Serve as a side dish or an appetizer dip. If served as a side dish, serve on a lettuce leaf. If served as an appetizer, place in a decorative serving bowl and serve with fresh vegetables or low-fat pita crisps or Melba rounds.

Skinny Secret

Enjoy with sliced veggies such as bell peppers, endive leaves, or slices of cucumber.

SERVES 4 AS A SIDE DISH, 12 AS AN APPETIZER DIP		CALORIES PER SERVING		NUTRITIONAL BREAKDOWN	
Serving size	½ cup, side dish; 2 tablespoons, appetizer	Original recipe	600	Fat	<1g
		SYS recipe	202	Carbohydrates	9g
				Protein	40g
				Sodium	421mg

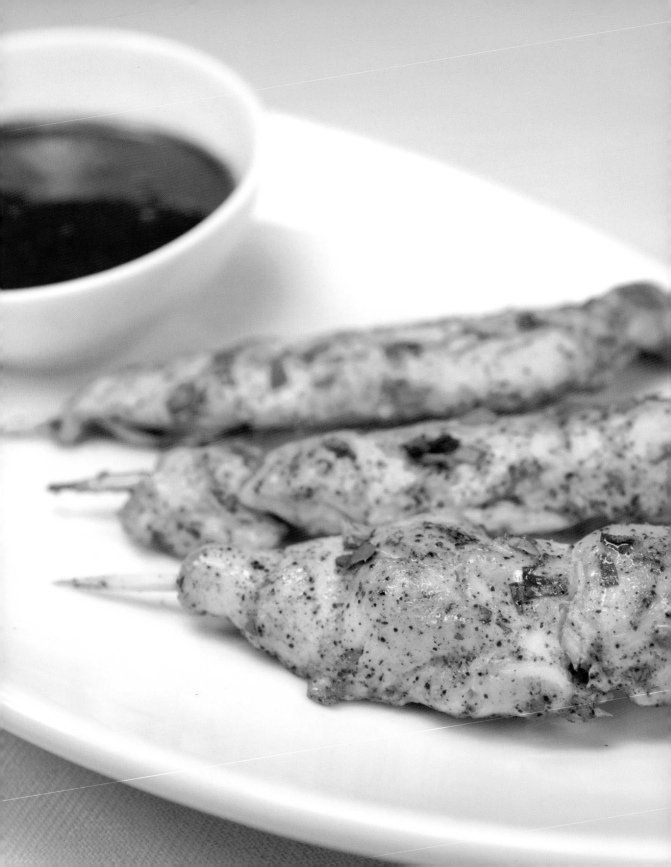

tasty chicken satay

Using a combination of Nutella and reduced-fat peanut butter saves over 500 calories and 35 grams of fat! This recipe can be made ahead of time, even grilling the chicken. To serve, bring sauce to room temperature and reheat chicken by throwing on a heated grill pan or grill for about a minute on each side.

¼ cup unsweetened coconut milk

¼ cup nonfat vanilla yogurt

1 tablespoon chopped fresh cilantro leaves

2 teaspoons curry powder

1 teaspoon chili powder

¼ cup peeled, seeded, and minced cucumber

1 pound boneless, skinless chicken breasts, sliced into ¼-inch-thick strips

15 (6-inch) bamboo skewers, soaked in water for 30 minutes

For the peanut sauce:

¼ cup Nutella

½ cup reduced-fat peanut butter

¼ cup low-sodium soy sauce

2 teaspoons chili powder

½ tablespoon dark brown sugar

1 tablespoon molasses

Juice of 2 limes

½ cup hot water

1 tablespoon chopped roasted peanuts, for garnish (optional)

1. In a large mixing bowl, combine the coconut milk, yogurt, cilantro, curry powder, chili powder, and cucumber. Mix to combine. Thread the chicken strips onto the soaked bamboo skewers. Place the skewers in the coconut mixture, coating on both sides. Cover and refrigerate for about 1 to 2 hours.

2. Make the peanut sauce by whisking together the Nutella, peanut butter, soy sauce, chili powder, sugar, molasses, lime juice, and water. Whisk well.

3. Preheat grill or grill pan to medium-high heat. Cook the chicken skewers for about 5 minutes on each side, brushing with marinade occasionally. Discard the remaining marinade.

4. Transfer the peanut sauce to a serving bowl. Top with chopped peanuts, if desired. Serve 1 skewer with 1 tablespoon of sauce.

MAKES APPROXIMATELY 15 SKEWERS		CALORIES PER SERVING		NUTRITIONAL BREAKDOWN	
Serving size	1 skewer	Original recipe	198	Fat	5g
		SYS recipe	113	Carbohydrates	34g
				Protein	10g
				Sodium	219mg

presto pesto dip

This pesto dip is spruced up with naturally low-calorie artichoke hearts. Plus, traditional high-fat olive oil and pine nuts are replaced with nonfat cream cheese, nonfat sour cream, and lemon juice. Two cups of traditional pesto can have more than 1,600 calories and over 20 grams of fat!

1 (8-ounce) package nonfat cream cheese

⅓ cup nonfat sour cream

1 (11-ounce) can artichoke hearts, drained and coarsely chopped

1 teaspoon lemon juice

1 tablespoon fresh basil leaves, coarsely chopped

2 tablespoons extra-virgin olive oil

¼ cup grated Parmesan cheese

Sea salt to taste

Black pepper to taste

Skinny Secret

Crisp, fresh basil is a key "bikini" ingredient. Fresh cilantro also works well in this recipe, as it's flavorful and virtually calorie-free.

1. In a food processor, combine the cream cheese, sour cream, artichoke hearts, lemon juice, basil, olive oil, and Parmesan. Purée until smooth and creamy, about 1 minute. Season with salt and pepper.

2. Transfer to a serving bowl and serve with fresh vegetables such as cucumber, jicama, and endive leaves. If you must have bread or chips, make sure they are low in fat by using Ak-mak crackers or baked pita crisps.

MAKES 2 CUPS	
Serving size	2 tablespoons

CALORIES PER SERVING	
Original recipe	410
SYS recipe	43

NUTRITIONAL BREAKDOWN	
Fat	4g
Carbohydrates	3g
Protein	3g
Sodium	34mg

deliciously skinny desserts

good bum brownies

Nonfat powdered milk is a perfect way to cut back on calories and fat and still maintain delicious milk flavor and texture. Use it not only for baking, but for your morning coffee too.

Nonstick cooking spray
4 eggs
⅓ cup granulated sugar
½ tablespoon butter
⅓ cup honey
2 teaspoons vanilla extract
¼ cup water
1½ cups plain flour
⅔ cup nonfat powdered milk
8 tablespoons cocoa powder
½ cup chopped pecans (optional)

Skinny Secret

Freeze leftover brownies for a low-cal, delicious snack and to help control portions.

1. Preheat oven to 350°F. Prepare a 9" × 13" baking dish by spraying with nonstick cooking spray.

2. In a mixing bowl, beat together the eggs, sugar, butter, and honey. Add the vanilla and water and mix well. Add the flour, powdered milk, and cocoa, and stir gently to combine, being careful not to overmix. Fold in the nuts, if using. Pour the mixture into the prepared dish and bake for 25 to 30 minutes. Undercooking is better than overcooking, so remove the brownies when the middle is still soft.

MAKES 24 BROWNIES	
Serving size	1 brownie

CALORIES PER SERVING	
Original recipe	243
SYS recipe	83

NUTRITIONAL BREAKDOWN	
Fat	3g
Carbohydrates	32g
Protein	4g
Sodium	30mg

wild about berries cheesecake

Omitting the butter and sugar in the crust and substituting ginger snaps saves more than 20 calories per serving. Whenever possible, skip on the butter and sugar to save calories in your everyday meals.

8 crushed ginger snaps

2 (8-ounce) packages nonfat cream cheese, softened

½ cup granulated sugar

2 tablespoons plain flour

1 teaspoon vanilla extract

Fine zest of ½ lemon

2 eggs

¼ cup nonfat milk

½ cup nonfat sour cream

1 cup fresh wild berries such as raspberries, blackberries, and blueberries, lightly crushed

1. Preheat oven to 350°F. Make the crust by sprinkling crushed ginger snaps into the bottom of an 8-inch springform pan. Set aside.

2. For the filling, combine the cream cheese, sugar, flour, vanilla, and lemon zest. Mix together well using a wooden spoon or electric mixer on medium speed. Once combined, mix in the eggs. Combine well. Add the milk and mix well. Pour into the prepared pan.

3. Bake for 40 to 50 minutes or until the center is nearly set when shaken.

4. Cool in the pan on a wire rack for about 15 minutes. Use a thin knife to loosen the cake from the sides of the pan. Remove the pan sides and let cool for 1 hour.

5. In a small mixing bowl, combine the sour cream and berries. Spread over the cheesecake. Loosely cover and chill for about 4 hours, or overnight.

SERVES 10		CALORIES PER SERVING		NUTRITIONAL BREAKDOWN	
Serving size	⅒ of cake	Original recipe	490	Fat	2g
		SYS recipe	105	Carbohydrates	12g
				Protein	9g
				Sodium	315mg

pecan delight

Sugar-free instant pudding mixes combined with nonfat milk make traditional desserts deliciously appealing to more health-conscious lives! Ginger snaps are also low in fat and high in flavor and a tasty alternative to traditional pie crusts.

1 (3.4-ounce) package sugar-free instant vanilla pudding mix
1¾ cups cold nonfat milk
4 thin ginger snap cookies
½ cup pecan halves, toasted

1. Whisk together the pudding mix and milk for 2 minutes in a medium mixing bowl. Refrigerate for 5 to 7 minutes.

2. Place the ginger snap cookies in the bottom of a sherbet dish, wine glass, or other decorative dessert dish. Spoon the pudding mixture over the top, and top with pecans.

To toast pecans: Place pecans in a dry skillet over medium-low heat. Toast until fragrant and lightly browned, shaking skillet occasionally to toast evenly and prevent burning, about 3 minutes.

Skinny Secret

Toasting the pecans brings out their nutty flavor, creating that traditional pecan pie taste without the traditional pecan pie calories!

SERVES 4	
Serving size	½ cup

CALORIES PER SERVING	
Original recipe	452
SYS recipe	189

NUTRITIONAL BREAKDOWN	
Fat	10g
Carbohydrates	19g
Protein	5g
Sodium	404mg

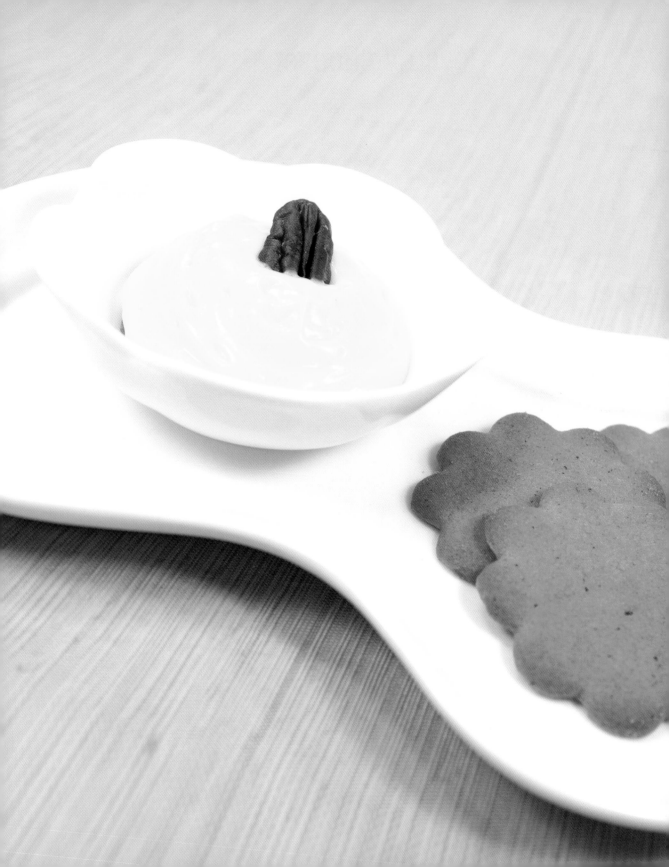

i love ny cheesecake

Using a combination of low-fat, nonfat, and high-fat ingredients is a good way to maintain flavor without sacrificing texture.

1 cup crushed graham crackers (about 20 squares)
3 tablespoons butter, melted
2 (8-ounce) packages nonfat cream cheese, softened
1 (8-ounce) package regular cream cheese, softened
½ cup plus 1 tablespoon granulated sugar
1 tablespoon plain flour
2 teaspoons vanilla extract
3 eggs
¼ cup nonfat milk

1. Preheat oven to 375°F. Prepare the crust by combining the graham cracker crumbs and butter in a mixing bowl. Grease the bottom of a springform pan and press the graham cracker mixture into the bottom of the pan. Let set in the refrigerator until ready to use.

2. In a large mixing bowl or standing mixer, beat together the cream cheese and sugar until well combined, about 3 minutes. Add the flour and vanilla. Mix well. Add the eggs one at a time, blending well. Add the milk and blend well.

3. Pour the mixture into the prepared pan. Bake for 55 to 60 minutes, until the center jiggles slightly when lightly shaken. Remove from the oven and set on a wire rack to cool for 15 minutes. Using a thin knife, loosen the edges of the cake from the pan. Let cool completely, about 1 hour. Remove the pan sides; cover and refrigerate for 4 hours or overnight.

SERVES 10		CALORIES PER SERVING		NUTRITIONAL BREAKDOWN	
Serving size	⅟₁₀ of cake	Original recipe	440	Fat	12g
		SYS recipe	218	Carbohydrates	21g
				Protein	10g
				Sodium	411mg

spiced carrot cake

The natural sweetness of the applesauce and pineapple make up for the flavor of sugar without the "empty" non-nutritious calories.

4 slices wheat bread, crumbled

4 eggs

4 tablespoons canola oil

2 teaspoons vanilla extract

1⅓ cup nonfat powdered milk

2 teaspoons baking soda

⅔ cup brown sugar

2 teaspoons ground cinnamon

1 pinch ground nutmeg

1 cup canned chopped pineapple, drained

1 cup applesauce

½ cup peeled and grated carrots

1. Preheat oven to 350°F. Spray a bundt-style cake pan with nonstick spray. In a blender or food processor, combine all the ingredients and process until smooth.

2. Pour the batter into the prepared cake pan and bake for 40 to 45 minutes or until a toothpick inserted comes out clean.

Skinny Secret

The natural sugars in the pineapple add to the depth of this recipe without overpowering sweetness.

SERVES 12	
Serving size	¹⁄₁₂ of cake

CALORIES PER SERVING	
Original recipe	740
SYS recipe	189

NUTRITIONAL BREAKDOWN	
Fat	2g
Carbohydrates	30g
Protein	6g
Sodium	127mg

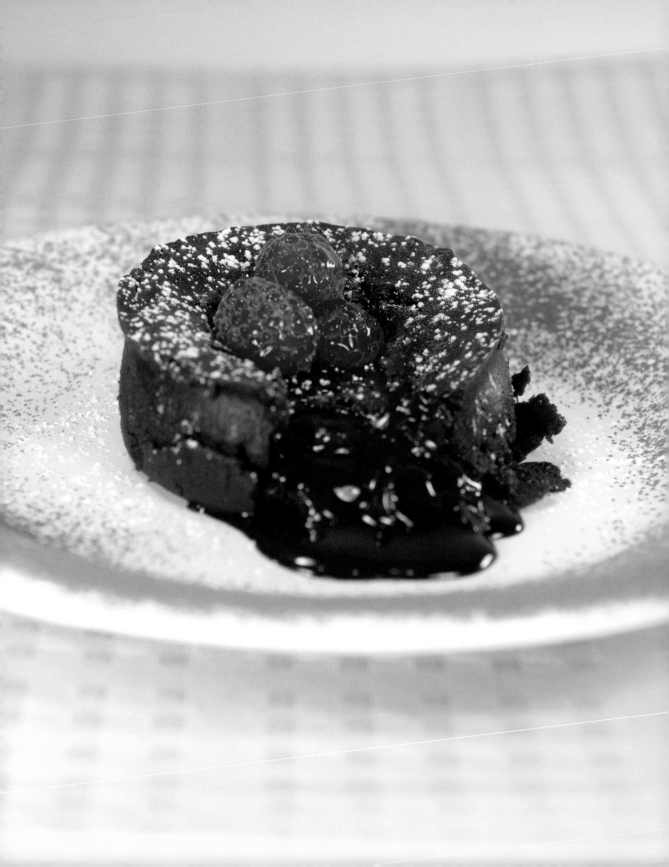

smitten for molten chocolate cake

Cutting back slightly on the amount of whipping cream and using fewer eggs are great ways to maintain flavor and texture without sacrificing the consistency of this dessert favorite.

6 tablespoons butter, plus extra for greasing

4 ounces semisweet chocolate

2 tablespoons whipping cream

2 tablespoons plain flour

1 teaspoon vanilla extract

2 eggs

2 egg yolks

2 tablespoons powdered sugar

1. Preheat oven to 400°F. Lightly grease 8 ramekins or custard cups with butter.

2. In the top of a double-boiler, combine the butter and chocolate, and heat until both are melted. Stir gently to combine. Stir in the whipping cream. Add the flour. Gently stir to combine.

3. In a medium mixing bowl, beat together the vanilla, eggs, egg yolks, and sugar until well combined and the mixture thickens, about 8 minutes. Using a rubber spatula, fold ⅓ of the egg mixture into the chocolate mixture until well blended. Repeat until all is combined.

4. Pour equal amounts of the mixture into each ramekin, filling about ¾ full. Bake for 7 to 8 minutes, until the edges are set and the center is jiggly.

Skinny Secret

Whenever possible, use dark baking chocolate for recipes. It has a higher cocoa content, rich chocolate flavor, and less sugar. As an added bonus, because it's rich in natural cocoa, it is more easily digested.

SERVES 8	
Serving size	1 mini-molten cake

CALORIES PER SERVING	
Original recipe	451
SYS recipe	191

NUTRITIONAL BREAKDOWN	
Fat	21g
Carbohydrates	11g
Protein	3g
Sodium	58mg

fudgy chocolate brownies

Coffee has a strong flavor that most people love, even in baked goods. Using it in this recipe is a perfect way to keep flavor high without adding any fat or calories. In addition, applesauce is naturally sweet and can be used to substitute for some or all of the sugar in recipes. Then, the egg whites help balance out the density of the applesauce, keeping your recipes lighter in texture.

Nonstick cooking spray
⅓ cup unsweetened cocoa
⅓ cup plain flour
1 teaspoon baking powder
¼ teaspoon baking soda
¼ teaspoon sea salt
⅔ cup granulated sugar
⅓ cup water
1 teaspoon instant coffee
⅓ cup applesauce
1 teaspoon vanilla extract
2 egg whites

Skinny Secret

You can also use coffee to flavor yogurt for a smoothie or to blend with ice for a quick, easy, low-cal granita.

1. Preheat oven to 350°F. Spray an 8-inch square baking dish with nonstick spray. In a mixing bowl, combine the cocoa, flour, baking powder, baking soda, salt, and sugar. Mix well.

2. In a small-quart boiler, bring the water to a boil. Remove from heat and add the coffee; stir to dissolve. In a small bowl, combine the applesauce, vanilla, and egg whites. Mix well. Add the coffee mixture and mix well. Pour the liquid mixture into the dry mixture and mix well.

3. Pour the mixture into the prepared dish. Bake for 30 minutes or until a toothpick inserted comes out clean. Let cool for 10 minutes, then run a knife around the edges to loosen. When cooled completely, slice into 2-inch squares and serve.

MAKES 16 BROWNIES	
Serving size	1 brownie

CALORIES PER SERVING	
Original recipe	243
SYS recipe	63

NUTRITIONAL BREAKDOWN	
Fat	.5g
Carbohydrates	14g
Protein	1g
Sodium	66mg

chipper chocolate chip cake

Cutting back on the oil and sugar used is a quick, simple way to cut calories without sacrificing flavor and texture. As well, using low-fat buttermilk and nonfat milk is an automatic calorie slimmer.

¾ cup canola oil

1½ cups granulated sugar

4 (1-ounce) squares unsweetened chocolate, melted and cooled slightly

3 teaspoons vanilla extract

5 eggs

2 cups plain flour

1 teaspoon baking soda

1 teaspoon sea salt

1 cup low-fat buttermilk

1¾ cups semisweet chocolate chips

For the frosting:

½ cup butter, softened

4 cups powdered sugar

¾ cup cocoa powder

⅔ cup nonfat milk

2 teaspoons vanilla extract

1. Preheat oven to 350°F. Line 3 (9-inch) round cake pans with parchment paper cut to fit the bottom of the pan. In a large mixing bowl, beat together the oil and sugar until somewhat light and fluffy. Add the chocolate and vanilla; mix well. Add the eggs one at a time, combining well after each addition. Separately, combine the flour, baking soda, and salt. Add the flour mixture and the buttermilk to the oil mixture a bit at a time, stirring until all the ingredients are incorporated. Fold in the chocolate chips.

2. Pour the batter into the prepared pans. Bake for 30 to 35 minutes, or until a toothpick inserted comes out clean. Cool on a wire rack for 10 minutes, then remove from the pan and allow to cool completely.

3. Make the frosting by creaming together the butter and 2 cups of the sugar in a large mixing bowl. Cream together until light and fluffy. Separately, combine the remaining sugar and cocoa powder. Mix well. Then, alternating, add some of the cocoa mixture, blend, then some of the milk, a little at a time. When all is combined, add the vanilla and beat well.

4. Spread some frosting on the top of each cake layer. Assemble the layers, and then spread frosting over the top and sides of the cake.

SERVES 20		CALORIES PER SERVING		NUTRITIONAL BREAKDOWN	
Serving size	¹⁄₂₀ of cake	Original recipe	648	Fat	17g
		SYS recipe	329	Carbohydrates	22g
				Protein	4g
				Sodium	53mg

date nut chews

The natural sugars in the fruit mean less sugar added to the recipe, translating to fewer calories and fat for you!

Nonstick cooking spray
1½ cups chopped pitted dates
½ cup raisins
1¼ cups water
6 tablespoons butter, cut into pieces
2 eggs
1 teaspoon vanilla extract
1 cup whole-wheat flour
1 teaspoon baking soda
5 teaspoons sugar substitute
½ teaspoon ground cinnamon
¼ teaspoon ground nutmeg
¼ teaspoon sea salt
¼ cup finely chopped walnuts (or substitute pecans, if preferred)

Skinny Secret

Whole-wheat flour is used here, making this dessert truly healthy with good fats, protein, and carbs. With this much nutrition, you may want to enjoy this dessert for breakfast!

1. Preheat oven to 350°F. Spray a 9" x 13" rectangular baking dish with nonstick spray. In large-quart boiler, heat the dates, raisins, and water over medium-high heat until boiling. Reduce heat and simmer, uncovered, until the dates and raisins are tender and the water is absorbed, about 10 minutes. Remove from heat and add the butter, stirring until melted; remove from heat and set aside to cool.

2. Once the date mixture has cooled, add the eggs and vanilla, and mix well. Add the flour, baking soda, sugar substitute, cinnamon, nutmeg, and salt. Spread the batter evenly into the prepared baking dish and sprinkle with walnuts.

3. Bake for 30 to 35 minutes, or until the cake springs back when lightly touched. Cool on a wire rack, and cut into squares.

MAKES 24 COOKIES		CALORIES PER SERVING		NUTRITIONAL BREAKDOWN	
Serving size	1 cookie	Original recipe	213	Fat	4g
		SYS recipe	65	Carbohydrates	8g
				Protein	10g
				Sodium	5mg

no more pounds pound cake

There are many variations on pound cake—some use sour cream, some buttermilk, and still others use cream cheese. Substituting applesauce gives a natural sweetness that is enhanced by the lemon zest. Add fresh berries when serving for a low-cal, low-fat alternative.

Nonstick cooking spray
¼ cup butter
⅔ cup granulated sugar
⅔ cup applesauce
fine zest of 1 lemon
1 teaspoon vanilla extract
1 egg
2 egg whites
1¾ cups plain flour
2 teaspoons baking powder
1 teaspoon sea salt
⅓ cup nonfat milk

1. Preheat oven to 350°F. Coat a 9" × 5" inch loaf pan with nonstick cooking spray. Using an electric mixer or standing mixer, beat together the butter and sugar. Add the applesauce, lemon, and vanilla; beat until well blended. Blend in the egg and egg whites.

2. In a separate bowl, sift together the flour, baking powder, and salt. With mixer on low, add ⅓ of the flour mixture to the applesauce mixture, then add half the milk; beat until well combined. Add another ⅓ of flour mixture, then add the rest of the milk, and beat until well combined. Add the remaining flour mixture and beat until all is incorporated. Do not overbeat.

3. Pour the batter into the prepared loaf pan and bake for 1 hour or until a toothpick inserted comes out clean. Allow to cool for 10 minutes. Use a thin knife to loosen the cake from the sides of the pan. Remove from the pan, slice, and serve.

Skinny Secret

Save your cake baking for large parties, when you won't be tempted afterward with lots of leftovers. While making the cake, clean your mixing bowls with a sponge, not your fingers!

SERVES 10	
Serving size	1/10 of cake

CALORIES PER SERVING	
Original recipe	430
SYS recipe	161

NUTRITIONAL BREAKDOWN	
Fat	18g
Carbohydrates	24g
Protein	4g
Sodium	51mg

very berry strawberry shortcake

Sugar-free strawberry preserves make a healthy and easy strawberry syrup for this super-low-cal yet satisfying shortcake.

1 package frozen biscuits such as Pillsbury
2 pints fresh strawberries, cleaned, trimmed, and sliced
1 (13.5-ounce) jar sugar-free strawberry preserves
1 can fat-free ready-made whipped cream

1. Preheat oven to 375°F. Place the biscuits on a baking sheet and bake for 16 to 20 minutes.

2. Remove from oven. For each serving, place the bottom half of a biscuit on a serving plate. Top with 1½ tablespoons fresh strawberries and 1½ tablespoons preserves, then add the top of the biscuit half. Top with an additional 1½ tablespoons fresh strawberries, and finish with 2 heaping tablespoons of whipped cream. Garnish with additional fresh strawberries if desired.

Skinny Secret

Try substituting your favorite berries and preserves such as raspberry, blackberry, or blueberry, in this recipe.

SERVES 12	
Serving size	1 biscuit with toppings

CALORIES PER SERVING	
Original recipe	561
SYS recipe	237

NUTRITIONAL BREAKDOWN	
Fat	9g
Carbohydrates	34g
Protein	.18g
Sodium	1,681mg

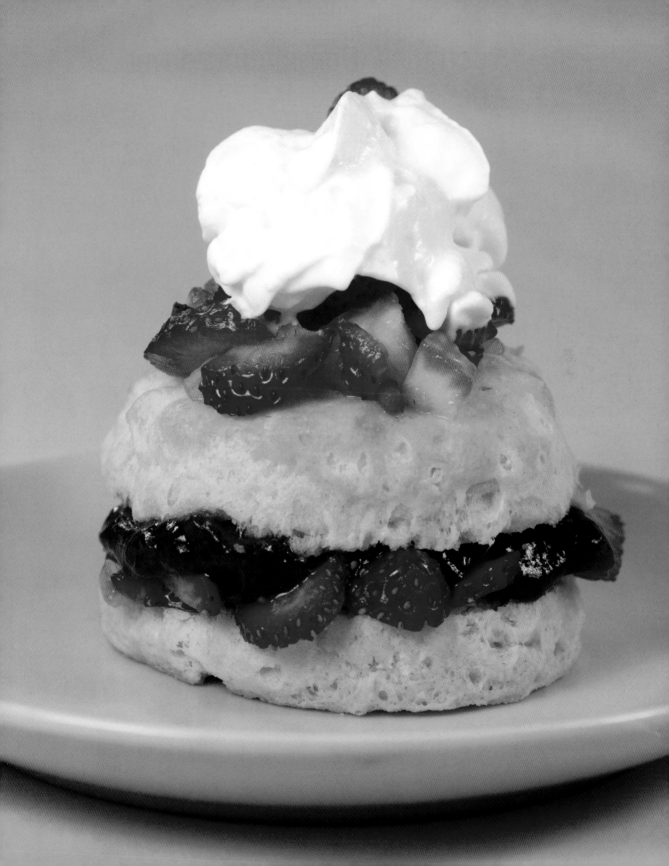

don't lay it on me four-layer dessert

Using sugar substitutes for baking is a great way to save on calories and fat. However, most substitutes taste sweeter than actual sugar, so you don't need to use as much.

Nonstick cooking spray

1 cup plain flour

1 stick butter, softened

½ cup chopped pecan halves

1 (8-ounce) package nonfat cream cheese

½ cup powdered sugar

¼ cup sugar substitute

1 (8-ounce) container fat-free Cool Whip or other whipped topping

2 (3.4-ounce) packages sugar-free instant chocolate pudding

3 cups nonfat milk

1. Preheat oven to 375°F. Lightly spray a 9" × 13" baking dish with nonstick spray. In a bowl, combine the flour, butter, and pecans. Mix well. Press the mixture into the bottom of the baking dish and bake for 15 minutes. Remove from the oven and allow to cool completely.

2. In a mixing bowl, mix together the cream cheese, sugar, sugar substitute, and 1 cup of the whipped topping. Mix together until well combined, and then spread over the baked crust.

3. Using an electric mixer or standing mixer, combine the pudding mix and milk. Beat on medium speed for 2 to 3 minutes until the mixture thickens. Spread on top of the cream cheese mixture.

4. Spread the remaining whipped topping on top of the pudding mixture. Cover and refrigerate for 4 hours or overnight. Slice into 2-inch squares and serve.

MAKES 32 SQUARES	
Serving size	1 square

CALORIES PER SERVING	
Original recipe	545
SYS recipe	77

NUTRITIONAL BREAKDOWN	
Fat	3g
Carbohydrates	10g
Protein	3g
Sodium	98mg

peanutty butter cookies

Sugar is often the real killer in desserts. Finding alternate ways to sweeten foods is key. Here, substitute apple juice concentrate and sugar substitute to keep calories and fat to a minimum.

1 cup creamy peanut butter

1 cup frozen apple juice concentrate, thawed, not diluted

½ cup sugar substitute

2 teaspoons vanilla extract

1 cup plain flour

1½ teaspoons baking soda

1. Preheat oven to 350°F. Line a baking sheet with parchment paper. In a mixing bowl, combine the peanut butter, juice concentrate, sugar substitute, and vanilla. Blend together well.

2. In a separate bowl, combine the flour and baking soda. Stir to combine and then stir into the peanut butter mixture until well combined.

3. Drop by teaspoonfuls onto the prepared baking sheet about 2 inches apart. Using a fork that has been dipped lightly in flour, gently press the tops of the cookie dough to flatten. Bake for about 10 minutes or until lightly browned. Remove from oven, cool on a wire rack, and serve.

Skinny Secret

These cookies make great little healthy snacks for both adults and kids. Keep some on hand in an airtight container to help with those sweet cravings. Just be sure to remember portion control! If they are too tempting to have around, share them with your neighbors.

MAKES 60 COOKIES	
Serving size	1 cookie

CALORIES PER SERVING	
Original recipe	135
SYS recipe	45

NUTRITIONAL BREAKDOWN	
Fat	2g
Carbohydrates	5g
Protein	1g
Sodium	45mg

fruitiest cobbler

Nonstick cooking spray keeps excess calories out of the dish and prevents your food from sticking. As well, to keep fat and calories to a minimum but flavor high, use a sugar substitute and sugar-free pie filling.

Nonstick cooking spray
1 cup butter
1 cup sugar substitute
4 eggs
1 teaspoon vanilla
2 cups plain flour
2 teaspoons baking powder
1 (20-ounce) can sugar-free blueberry pie filling

Skinny Secret

Add fresh blueberries when serving for extra flavor and color!

1. Preheat oven to 350°F. Spray a 9" × 13" baking pan with nonstick spray. In a large mixing bowl, combine the butter and sugar substitute. Add the eggs and mix until well blended using a wooden spoon or electric mixer. Add the vanilla, and mix well.

2. Separately, in small mixing bowl, combine the flour and baking powder and stir to blend. Stir the flour mixture into the butter mixture and mix well. Pour the mixture into the prepared baking pan. Spoon the pie filling onto the mixture in spoonfuls, spacing evenly over entire dish.

3. Bake for 45 to 50 minutes. (The filling will sink into the cake.) Serve bottom side up.

SERVES 12	
Serving size	1/12 of cobbler

CALORIES PER SERVING	
Original recipe	622
SYS recipe	324

NUTRITIONAL BREAKDOWN	
Fat	17g
Carbohydrates	36g
Protein	4g
Sodium	132mg

peachy keen crumble

Cutting back on sugar and butter helps keep away calories, but using reduced-fat Bisquick baking mix is key!

Nonstick cooking spray
8 ripe peaches, peeled, pitted, and sliced
Juice of 1 lemon
1 pinch ground cinnamon
1 pinch ground nutmeg
½ cup reduced-fat Bisquick baking mix
2 tablespoons dark brown sugar
2 tablespoons butter, cut into small cubes
¼ cup quick-cooking oats

1. Preheat oven to 375°F. Lightly coat a 9-inch pie pan with nonstick cooking spray. In a small mixing bowl, toss the peaches with the lemon juice, cinnamon, and nutmeg. Separately, combine the Bisquick and brown sugar. Using your fingers, crumble the butter into the Bisquick mixture. Add the oats and mix well. Sprinkle the Bisquick mixture on top of the peaches.

2. Bake until the peaches are soft and the topping is browned, about 30 minutes. Cut into 12 slices and serve.

Skinny Secret

This delicious dessert is simple to make—so simple you can make it in individual ramekins for a quick, easy, low-fat dessert any day of the week.

SERVES 12	
Serving size	¹⁄₁₂ of pie

CALORIES PER SERVING	
Original recipe	300
SYS recipe	93

NUTRITIONAL BREAKDOWN	
Fat	3g
Carbohydrates	26g
Protein	2g
Sodium	40mg

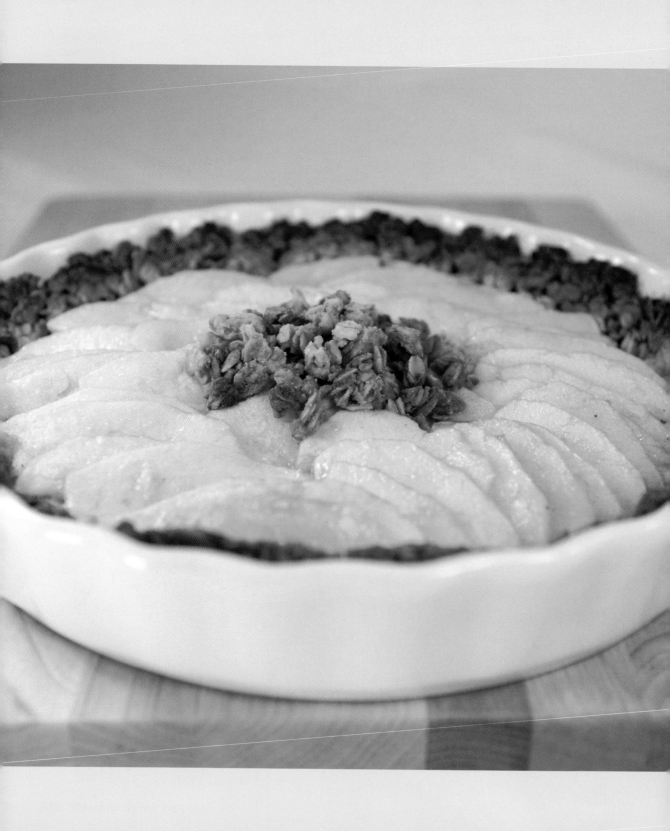

apple pie

Substituting honey is a great way to sweeten a recipe with a natural sugar. However, use it in moderation because honey is not as low in calories as you may think!

Nonstick cooking spray
⅓ cup butter
1 tablespoon honey
2 tablespoons plain flour
1 cup rolled oats
4 cups Golden Delicious apples, peeled and thinly sliced
Fine zest of ½ lemon
Juice of ½ lemon
2 tablespoons plain flour
¼ cup honey

1. Preheat oven to 350°F. Spray a 9-inch pie pan with nonstick cooking spray. In a small mixing bowl, use a fork to combine the butter and honey. Mix in the flour and oats. Combine well to make a dough. Dip your fingers in the flour and then press the dough into the bottom and up the sides of the prepared pie pan. Bake for 10 minutes. Remove from the oven and set aside to cool.

2. Prepare the filling by tossing the apples in a medium mixing bowl with the lemon zest, juice, flour, and honey. Arrange the coated apple slices in the pie pan. Cover with aluminum foil and bake for 35 minutes. Remove the foil and bake for an additional 10 minutes.

Skinny Secret

Lemon juice not only helps to prevent the apples from turning brown during preparation but also adds flavor.

SERVES 10	
Serving size	⅒ of pie

CALORIES PER SERVING	
Original recipe	280
SYS recipe	164

NUTRITIONAL BREAKDOWN	
Fat	7g
Carbohydrates	18g
Protein	11g
Sodium	2mg

smart tart wild berry tart

Wild berries are a nutritious and colorful way to enjoy great flavor with minimal calories. Using ginger snaps and low-fat cheese keep flavor in and calories out.

Nonstick cooking spray

1½ cups crushed ginger snap cookies

2 tablespoons granulated sugar

1 pinch sea salt

2 tablespoons butter, melted

1 egg white, beaten

3 cups reduced-fat ricotta cheese

4 tablespoons honey

Fine zest of 1 orange

Fine zest of 1 lemon

2 teaspoons vanilla extract

1 cup fresh strawberries, cleaned and trimmed

1 cup fresh raspberries

1 cup fresh blueberries

1 cup fresh blackberries

1. Preheat oven to 350°F. Spray a 10-inch tart pan with a removable bottom with nonstick cooking spray. Combine the ginger snaps, sugar, and salt in a medium mixing bowl. Add the butter and egg white, and mix until well combined. Press the mixture into the bottom of the tart pan and bake for 15 to 20 minutes, or until the crust is dry. Remove from the oven and set aside to cool completely.

2. In a mixing bowl, combine the ricotta, 2 tablespoons of the honey, orange and lemon zest, and vanilla using a wire whisk or electric mixer. Refrigerate the mixture for at least 30 minutes. Pour the mixture into the tart pan and refrigerate for 1 hour or more. Top with the berries, drizzle with the remaining honey, and serve.

SERVES 10		CALORIES PER SERVING		NUTRITIONAL BREAKDOWN	
Serving size	⅒ of tart	Original recipe	310	Fat	7g
		SYS recipe	218	Carbohydrates	41g
				Protein	16g
				Sodium	175mg

oaty oatmeal cookies

Naturally sweet applesauce and low-calorie, light egg whites are key to this lower-calorie version of a traditional favorite.

1 cup plain flour
1 cup quick-cooking oats
½ teaspoon baking powder
½ teaspoon baking soda
½ teaspoon sea salt
1 pinch ground cinnamon
1 pinch ground nutmeg
2 egg whites
½ cup applesauce
⅓ cup honey
1 teaspoon vanilla extract
⅓ cup raisins

1. Preheat oven to 375°F. Line a baking sheet with parchment paper or spray with nonstick cooking spray. In a medium mixing bowl, combine the flour, oats, baking powder, baking soda, salt, cinnamon, and nutmeg. Mix well. Add the egg whites, applesauce, honey, and vanilla, and stir to combine. Add the raisins and mix well.

2. Drop by heaping teaspoonfuls onto the prepared baking sheet about 2 inches apart. Bake for 8 to 10 minutes, until lightly browned.

Skinny Secret

Oatmeal is high in fiber and therefore filling, making these cookies perfect for a light dessert or as a snack.

MAKES 32 COOKIES	
Serving size	1 cookie

CALORIES PER SERVING	
Original recipe	80
SYS recipe	38

NUTRITIONAL BREAKDOWN	
Fat	.4g
Carbohydrates	9g
Protein	1g
Sodium	6mg

tropi-low-cal granita

Granitas are typically filled with sugar. A hint of powdered sugar along with refreshing citrus and effervescent Sierra Mist Free are all great ways to make this dessert lively and nearly calorie-free.

2 cups blueberries

1 cup strawberries, cleaned and trimmed

2 tablespoons powdered sugar

Fine zest of ½ lemon

Juice of ½ lemon

Fine zest of ½ lime

Juice of ½ lime

3 cups Sierra Mist Free

Skinny Secret

Granitas are a refreshing way to curb your sweet tooth without breaking your calorie bank. Keep some in the freezer for quick, light snacks.

1. Process the blueberries and strawberries with the sugar in a food processor until smooth. Add the lemon zest and juice and lime zest and juice, and process until smooth. Pour the mixture into an 11" × 7" dish, and stir in the Sierra Mist. Cover and freeze for about 8 hours. Remove from the freezer and let stand for 5 minutes.

2. Chop the mixture into large chunks and place in a food processor in batches, pulsing 5 to 6 times. Serve immediately in martini or wine glasses. Garnish with additional lemon or lime zest if desired.

SERVES 8		CALORIES PER SERVING		NUTRITIONAL BREAKDOWN	
Serving size	1 cup	Original recipe	124	Fat	.17g
		SYS recipe	20	Carbohydrates	9g
				Protein	.4g
				Sodium	10mg

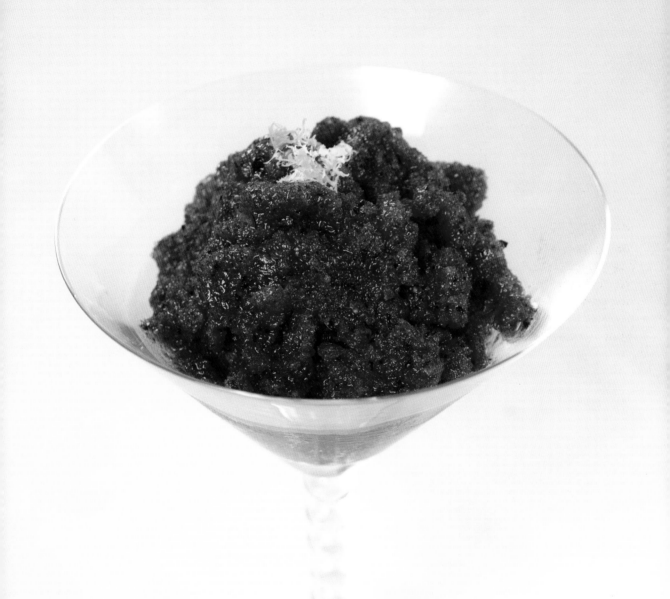

peanut butter chocolate bars

Sugar substitute, nonfat milk, and healthier Nutella all contribute to making these bars deliciously low-calorie.

Nonstick cooking spray
1 stick butter, softened
1 cup sugar substitute
⅓ cup brown sugar
½ cup nonfat milk
½ cup creamy peanut butter
1 egg
1 teaspoon vanilla extract
1 cup plain flour
1 cup quick-cooking oats
½ teaspoon baking soda
¼ teaspoon sea salt
¾ cup Nutella

Skinny Secret

Nutella is a chocolate-hazelnut blend made with skim milk and cocoa. It is lower in fat than peanut butter but has plenty of flavor. Use it in all types of recipes including breakfasts, appetizers, and snacks.

1. Preheat oven to 350°F. Spray a 13" × 9" baking dish with nonstick cooking spray. In a standing mixer or using a handheld electric mixer, beat together the butter, sugar substitute, and brown sugar until well combined. Add the milk, peanut butter, egg, and vanilla, and blend.

2. In a small mixing bowl, stir together the flour, oats, baking soda, and salt until blended. Gradually mix the flour mixture into the butter mixture. Once combined, mix in the Nutella until well combined.

3. Pour the mixture into the prepared baking dish and spread out evenly. Bake for 20 to 22 minutes. Cool completely on a wire rack. Cut into squares and serve.

MAKES 48 BARS		CALORIES PER SERVING		NUTRITIONAL BREAKDOWN	
Serving size	1 bar	Original recipe	590	Fat	1g
		SYS recipe	62	Carbohydrates	2g
				Protein	1g
				Sodium	13mg

not your grandma's custard éclair

This recipe proves éclairs don't have to be completely fattening. Egg substitutes such as Egg Beaters, sugar-free pudding mix, nonfat milk, nonfat cream cheese, and nonfat whipped topping are combined to tantalize your taste buds without overloading on fat.

1 cup water
½ cup (1 stick) butter
1 cup plain flour
1 (8-ounce) container Egg Beaters Original egg substitute
2 (3.4-ounce) packages sugar-free vanilla instant pudding mix
3 cups nonfat milk
1 (8-ounce) package nonfat cream cheese
1 (12-ounce) container fat-free whipped topping, such as Cool Whip
2 tablespoons chocolate syrup (for drizzling)

1. Preheat oven to 400°F. In a small boiler over medium heat, bring the water and butter to a boil. Stir in the flour until it forms into a ball. Remove from heat and gradually stir in the Egg Beaters. Spread the mixture into a jellyroll pan. Bake for 30 minutes.

2. In a large mixing bowl or standing mixer, beat together the pudding mix and milk until the mixture is well blended and thickened. Blend in the cream cheese until well combined. Spread the cream cheese mixture over the cooled cake. Spread the whipped topping over the pudding mixture. Drizzle the chocolate syrup over the top. Chill for 1 hour or more, and serve cold.

Skinny Secret

Egg Beaters are called an egg substitute but they are actually real egg whites to which vitamins and nutrients have been added. If you prefer, just use egg whites.

SERVES 12		CALORIES PER SERVING		NUTRITIONAL BREAKDOWN	
Serving size	1 éclair	Original recipe	298	Fat	8g
		SYS recipe	225	Carbohydrates	25g
				Protein	8g
				Sodium	715mg

lemon lovers' lemon cake

Lighter than traditional cakes such as pound cake, angel food cake is virtually fat-free and is perfect for soaking up other flavors of fruits, juices, and filling, such as the lemon pie filling here.

1 angel food cake
1 (3.4-ounce) package sugar-free lemon pudding and pie filling
2 egg yolks
¼ cup granulated sugar
2¼ cups water

Skinny Secret

Lemon pudding and pie filling is different from the pudding mix! It's the perfect nonfat, low-calorie alternative for pies, glazes, and cakes.

Poke holes in the angel food cake. In a medium-quart boiler over medium heat, combine the pie filling mix, eggs, sugar, and ¼ cup of the water. Mix together, then stir in the remaining 2 cups water. Stir constantly with a wire whisk until the mixture comes to a full boil. Continue stirring and remove from heat. Pour the mixture over the cake. Serve warm or at room temperature.

SERVES 12		CALORIES PER SERVING		NUTRITIONAL BREAKDOWN	
Serving size	¹⁄₁₂ of cake	Original recipe	344	Fat	2g
		SYS recipe	157	Carbohydrates	24g
				Protein	4g
				Sodium	348mg

lime tart

Nonfat dry powdered milk is a great way to create your own healthful version of condensed milk. Other ways to cut down on calories and fat are to use a sugar substitute, sugar-free flavored gelatin, and nonfat sour cream.

½ cup plus ¾ cup water
1⅓ cup nonfat dry powdered milk
½ cup sugar substitute
1 (9-inch) pie shell
1 (3-ounce) package sugar-free lime-flavored gelatin mix
Fine zest of 1 lime
½ cup fresh lime juice
1 cup nonfat sour cream

1. Preheat oven to 350°F. Make the condensed milk by heating ½ cup of the water in a small-quart boiler. Stir in the powdered milk until it becomes a paste. Heat until hot, but not boiling. Stir in the sugar substitute. Heat for about 1 minute. Remove from heat and set aside.

2. Remove 1 pie shell from the package and bake for 10 minutes. Remove from oven and set aside to cool.

3. In a separate small-quart boiler, bring the remaining ¾ cup water to a boil and add the gelatin, stirring to dissolve. Remove from heat and let cool for about 5 minutes. Transfer the mixture to the refrigerator and let chill until it begins to congeal, about 30 minutes.

4. In a mixing bowl, combine the milk mixture, lime zest, and lime juice. Stir until blended. Stir in the sour cream, and then fold in the thickened gelatin. Pour the mixture into the pastry shell. Chill until firm, and serve.

Skinny Secret

For an even lighter but still refreshing dessert, skip the pie crust and serve the congealed lime mixture in martini or sherbet glasses. Add a slice of fresh lime for fun!

SERVES 10		CALORIES PER SERVING		NUTRITIONAL BREAKDOWN	
Serving size	⅒ of tart	Original recipe	401	Fat	1g
		SYS recipe	52	Carbohydrates	10g
				Protein	10g
				Sodium	99mg

berry berry strawberry cake

Using sugar-free strawberry gelatin adds extra strawberry flavor without adding the unwanted fat and calories. Frozen and fresh strawberries top off this fantastic strawberry dessert, which keeps fat and calories down by using egg whites and sugar substitutes.

Nonstick cooking spray

4 egg whites

1 package white cake mix

1 (3-ounce) package sugar-free strawberry-flavored gelatin

½ cup canola oil

½ cup water

½ can unsweetened frozen strawberries, thawed with juice

For the icing:

5 tablespoons plus 1 teaspoon butter

½ pint fresh strawberries, cleaned and trimmed

¾ cup powdered sugar

1 cup sugar substitute

1. Preheat oven to 350°F. Spray an 8- or 9-inch round cake pan with nonstick spray. In a medium mixing bowl, beat the egg whites for 2 minutes using an electric mixer or a standing mixer on medium speed. Add the cake mix, gelatin, oil, and water. Beat until well blended. Add the strawberries with juice. Blend well. Pour the mixture into the prepared cake pan and bake for 30 minutes.

2. Make the icing: Blend the butter with the strawberries. Add the powdered sugar and sugar substitute, and gently mix well. Spread over the slightly cooled cake.

SERVES 12	
Serving size	½₂ of cake

CALORIES PER SERVING	
Original recipe	393
SYS recipe	322

NUTRITIONAL BREAKDOWN	
Fat	19g
Carbohydrates	12g
Protein	2g
Sodium	300mg

banana-rama banana pudding cake

Substituting is easy in this delicious banana cake. Use nonfat milk instead of whole, sugar-free pudding and pie mix instead of regular, reduced-fat vanilla wafers instead of regular, and fat-free whipped topping.

3 cups nonfat milk

2 (3.4-ounce) packages sugar-free vanilla instant pudding and pie filling

30 reduced-fat vanilla wafers

3 medium bananas, sliced

1 (8-ounce) container fat-free whipped topping, such as Cool Whip

1. In a large mixing bowl, whisk together the milk and pudding mix for about 2 minutes, or until well blended. Let stand for about 5 minutes.

2. Arrange half of the wafers on the bottom and around the sides in one to two layers of a 2-quart baking dish or decorative casserole-style bowl. Add layers of half the bananas and half the pudding mixture, and repeat until all bananas and pudding are used. Once layers are completed, slide remaining wafers down sides of dish. Spread the whipped topping over the pudding. Refrigerate for 3 hours, or until ready to serve.

Skinny Secret

For a lighter banana pudding, skip the wafers and layer the pudding and bananas in a parfait glass and top with whipped cream.

SERVES 14		
Serving size	²/₃ cup	

CALORIES PER SERVING	
Original recipe	454
SYS recipe	188

NUTRITIONAL BREAKDOWN	
Fat	5g
Carbohydrates	35g
Protein	2g
Sodium	579mg

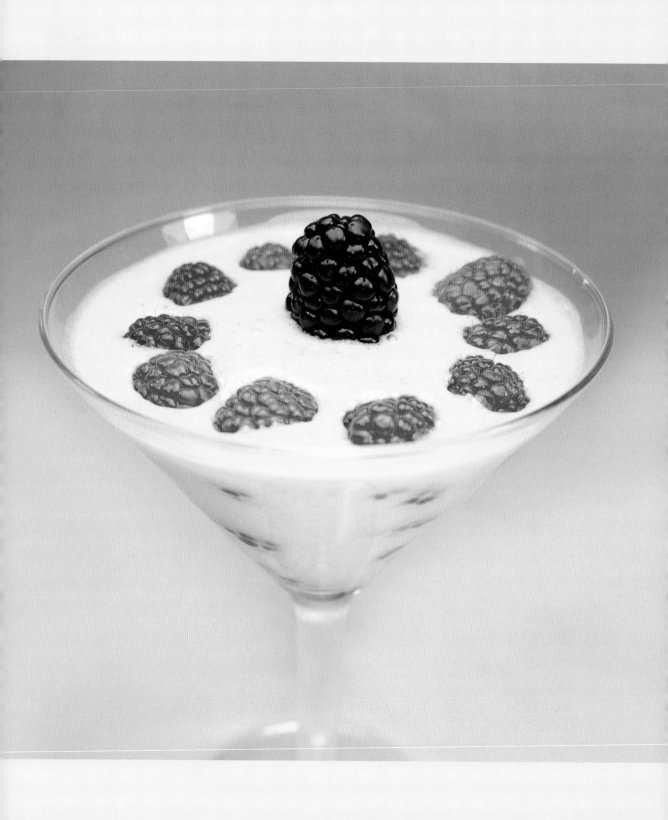

lovely lemon custard with fresh wild berries

Similar lemon desserts use heavy whipping cream and loads of sugar. Cutting back on the sugar and adding the flavors of lemon and Marsala make this a must-have dessert, especially with the natural sweetness of fresh berries.

6 egg yolks
½ tablespoon cold water
¼ cup granulated sugar
½ teaspoon sea salt
½ tablespoon fresh lemon juice
1 teaspoon fresh lemon zest
¼ cup Marsala wine
1 pint fresh raspberries
1 pint fresh blackberries

In a double-boiler, beat the egg yolks together with the water using a hand mixer (preferred) or wire whisk until they are foamy and light. Whisk in the sugar, salt, lemon juice, zest, and wine. Beat over hot, but not boiling, water until thickened and fluffy. Spoon into martini glasses and top with the berries. Serve warm.

Skinny Secret

Serving desserts in martini glasses or other individual-sized serving dishes helps curb the urge to go for second helpings!

SERVES 6	
Serving size	½ cup

CALORIES PER SERVING	
Original recipe	350
SYS recipe	158

NUTRITIONAL BREAKDOWN	
Fat	4g
Carbohydrates	22g
Protein	4g
Sodium	3mg

plum good crumble

Usually this type of crumble includes more sugar, lots of butter, and often, sour cream. Cutting back on the sugar and substituting applesauce keeps the flavor and texture and helps keep your figure slim and trim.

Nonstick cooking spray
3 pounds plums, pitted and thinly sliced
1 tablespoon fresh lemon juice
¼ cup light brown sugar
1 cup quick-cooking oats
⅓ cup plain flour
1 pinch ground cinnamon
4 tablespoons applesauce

1. Preheat oven to 400°F. Spray a 2-quart baking dish with nonstick spray. In separate medium mixing bowl, combine the plums and lemon juice and toss to coat. Add plum mixture to prepared baking dish. In a medium mixing bowl, combine the sugar, oats, flour, and cinnamon. Toss to combine. Add the applesauce, and use your fingers to toss the mixture until it resembles coarse crumbles. Sprinkle the oat topping over the plum mixture.

2. Bake for 25 to 30 minutes, until the plums are tender and the topping is lightly browned. Cool on a wire rack for 10 minutes and serve, or cool completely and serve later.

SERVES 12	
Serving size	½ of crumble

CALORIES PER SERVING	
Original recipe	340
SYS recipe	120

NUTRITIONAL BREAKDOWN	
Fat	1g
Carbohydrates	26g
Protein	3g
Sodium	2mg

decadent chocolate torte

Most of your calorie savings comes from using cocoa powder, reduced amounts of sugar, incorporating egg whites along with the egg yolks, and using nonstick spray instead of coating the pan with butter and flour. This is a truly delicious chocolate dessert not to be missed.

Nonstick cooking spray

3 ounces dark chocolate, chopped

½ cup cocoa powder

½ cup granulated sugar

½ cup boiling water

2 egg yolks

4 egg whites

3 tablespoons plain flour

1. Preheat oven to 375°F. Spray an 8-inch springform cake pan with nonstick spray. In a large mixing bowl, combine the chocolate, cocoa, and sugar, and stir to mix. Pour in the boiling water and whisk until the mixture is smooth and the chocolate is melted. In small bowl, whisk together the egg yolks and flour. Quickly whisk the egg yolk mixture into the chocolate and set aside.

2. Separately, in a medium mixing bowl, beat the egg whites with an electric mixer on high speed until soft peaks form. Gently fold the egg whites into the chocolate mixture until combined. Pour the mixture into the prepared cake pan.

3. Bake for 30 to 35 minutes or until a toothpick inserted comes out slightly wet. Remove from oven and set on a wire rack to cool. (The torte will sink in the center.) Once cooled, slice and serve.

Skinny Secret

This rich torte is so satisfying that up to 16 portions can actually be served, making each portion very bikini friendly.

SERVES 10	
Serving size	⅒ of torte

CALORIES PER SERVING	
Original recipe	480
SYS recipe	111

NUTRITIONAL BREAKDOWN	
Fat	7g
Carbohydrates	14g
Protein	5g
Sodium	32mg

tiramisu loves you

Enjoy this light version of this Italian favorite by using egg substitute, sugar substitute, nonfat cream cheese, fat-free whipped topping, and fat-free pound cake. Trust me, the yummy flavor will be no substitute!

¼ cup Egg Beaters Original or other egg substitute
½ cup granulated sugar
¼ cup sugar substitute
1½ teaspoons vanilla extract
1 (8-ounce) package nonfat cream cheese, cubed
1 (8-ounce) package fat-free whipped topping
1 tablespoon instant espresso powder
¼ cup hot water
1 cup cold water
1 fat-free loaf pound cake, cut into ½-inch slices
8 ounces semisweet chocolate, finely chopped

Skinny Secret

When serving this recipe, make sure to measure out servings into individual bowls. This recipe tastes so good you'll never know it was made with fat-free ingredients and you will for sure be tempted to indulge.

1. In a food processor, blend together the Egg Beaters and sugars until combined. Add the vanilla and process for about 1 minute. Add the cream cheese a little at a time and process until smooth. Transfer to a medium bowl. Cover and refrigerate for 1 hour.

2. Fold the whipped topping into the cream cheese mixture. In a shallow dish, dissolve the espresso powder in the hot water. Once dissolved, add the cold water.

3. Working quickly, dip the cake slices into the espresso liquid, coating both sides. Arrange the slices in the bottom of 13" × 9" baking dish, and smooth out with your fingers to mold the cake slices together. Sprinkle with half the chopped chocolate. Top with the cream cheese mixture, and sprinkle with the remaining chocolate. Cover and refrigerate for at least 3 hours or overnight before serving. Keep leftovers, if any, in the refrigerator.

SERVES 10		CALORIES PER SERVING		NUTRITIONAL BREAKDOWN	
Serving size	¹⁄₁₀ of "pie"	Original recipe	470	Fat	7g
		SYS recipe	276	Carbohydrates	43g
				Protein	5g
				Sodium	265mg

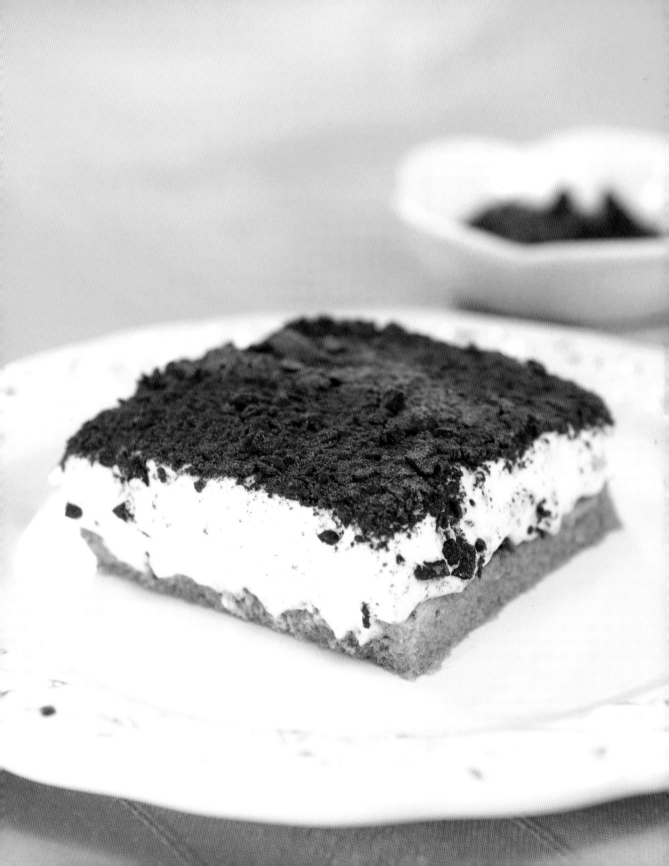

lazy day lemonade freeze

Making your own sugar-free condensed milk, as here in this recipe, saves a ton of calories and is worth the little extra effort.

1 teaspoon cornstarch
1 tablespoon cold water
1¼ cups dry nonfat powdered milk
½ cup water
½ cup sugar substitute
1 teaspoon vanilla extract
1 (6-ounce) can frozen lemonade concentrate, thawed
1 (8-ounce) container fat-free whipped topping
Juice of 1 lemon
10 reduced-fat vanilla wafer cookies, crushed

Skinny Secret

This delicious dessert is also perfect as a quick, light snack!

1. In a small bowl, combine the cornstarch and cold water. Mix together until the cornstarch is dissolved. In a microwave-safe dish, stir together the powdered milk and ½ cup water. Cover and microwave on high for 45 seconds. Stir the cornstarch mixture into the powdered milk mixture and microwave for 10 seconds, until thick. Stir in the sugar substitute and vanilla until well combined. Chill for 2 hours before using.

2. In a medium mixing bowl, combine the lemonade, whipped topping, chilled milk mixture, and the lemon juice. Stir until blended.

3. Divide the lemonade mixture into 10 ramekins and top with crushed cookies. Place in the freezer for at least 1 hour, or until ready to serve.

SERVES 10		CALORIES PER SERVING		NUTRITIONAL BREAKDOWN	
Serving size	½ cup plus 1 wafer	Original recipe	506	Fat	2g
		SYS recipe	87	Carbohydrates	18g
				Protein	1g
				Sodium	18mg

creamy chocolate pudding

Substituting nonfat vanilla yogurt is a great way to reduce calories, maximize flavor, and add a little extra protein in your diet.

1 (3.4-ounce) package sugar-free chocolate pudding mix
1½ cups nonfat milk
½ teaspoon Grand Marnier
1 egg white
2 teaspoons granulated sugar
4 tablespoons nonfat vanilla yogurt

1. In a small boiler over medium heat, stir together the pudding mix and milk, and bring to just before a boil, but do not boil. Continue stirring until the mixture is thickened. Stir in the Grand Marnier. Set aside.

2. Using an electric mixer, beat together the egg white and sugar until stiff peaks form. Fold into the pudding until all is combined. Spoon into 4 dessert dishes and chill. Serve with 1 tablespoon nonfat vanilla yogurt on top.

Skinny Secret

Don't be afraid to use liqueurs when cooking. They enhance the flavor of foods and the alcohol cooks out.

SERVES 4	
Serving size	½ cup

CALORIES PER SERVING	
Original recipe	299
SYS recipe	126

NUTRITIONAL BREAKDOWN	
Fat	.6g
Carbohydrates	16g
Protein	2g
Sodium	172mg

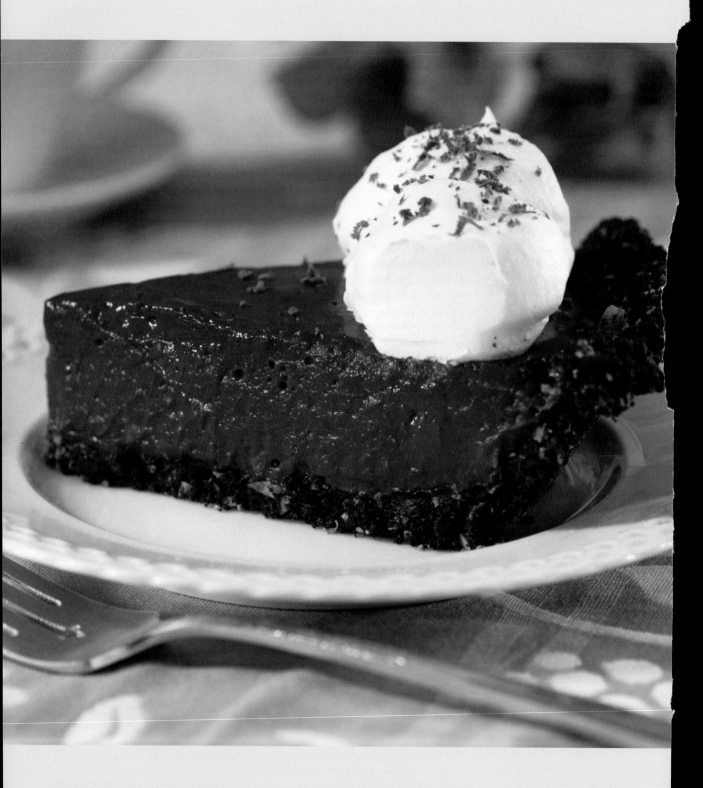

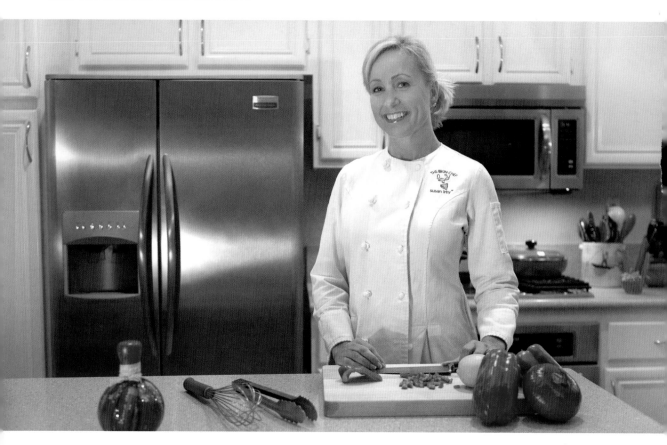

about the author

CHEF SUSAN IRBY has worked with multiple Master Chefs including George McNeill, Todd English, and Ming Tsai. Known as the Bikini Chef, specializing in "figure-flattering flavors," Chef Susan is host of *The Bikini Lifestyle with Susan Irby The Bikini Chef* on KFWB News Talk 980 in Los Angeles and author of *The $7 a Meal Quick & Easy Cookbook, The $7 a Meal Healthy Cookbook,* and *Cooking with Susan.* She has cooked for several celebrities including Patrick Swayze, David Spade, Kate Sagal, and Bill Handel, and appeared on *The Patti Gribow Show* and KLAC Los Angeles and numerous other media outlets. She lives in Orange County, CA. *Visit www.susanirby.com.*

mad 4 mud pie

Reduced-fat is the name of the game for this usually super-high-calorie, high-fat dessert. Use reduced-fat Oreo cookies, nonfat milk, fat-free whipped topping, and nonfat cream cheese to get the decadence you love without the calories you don't.

48 reduced-fat Oreo cookies
2 tablespoons butter, melted
½ cup nonfat milk
¼ cup (½ stick) butter
12 ounces semisweet chocolate chips
16 ounces fat-free whipped topping
1 (8-ounce) package nonfat cream cheese

1. Preheat oven to 350°F. In a food processor, grind 20 of the cookies with the 2 tablespoons melted butter. Press into the bottom and halfway up the sides of a 10-inch springform pan. Bake the crust for 10 minutes. Remove from oven, let cool slightly, and then chill in the refrigerator.

2. Make the filling: In a medium-quart boiler over medium heat, combine the milk, butter, and chocolate chips. Heat until the chocolate is just melted, but do not overheat or allow to boil. Stir together until completely smooth. Remove from heat and allow to cool slightly.

3. Grind 20 more of the Oreos in a food processor. In a separate bowl, combine the whipped topping and cream cheese. Mix well. Fold in ¾ of the cream cheese mixture with the ground Oreos. Spread into the chilled crust. Then, top with chocolate mixture. Chill about 30 minutes. Top the pie with dollops of remaining cream cheese. Break up the remaining Oreos and place on top of the cream cheese dollops. Freeze for about 1 hour before serving.

Skinny Secret

Even with all this yummy flavor, this recipe has half the fat and calories of the original! And the best part is that you can keep it in the freezer for up to 1 month.

SERVES 12	
Serving size	1/12 of pie

CALORIES PER SERVING	
Original recipe	680
SYS recipe	384

NUTRITIONAL BREAKDOWN	
Fat	24g
Carbohydrates	72g
Protein	5g
Sodium	123mg

index